FITNESS PROFESSIONALS

# EXERCISE IN WATER

complete guide to planning and instruction

rd edition

EBBIE LAWRENCE

A & C BLACK · LONDON

Published by A & C Black Publishers Ltd
38 Soho Square, London W1D 3HB
www.acblack.com

Third edition 2008
Second edition 2004
First edition 1998

ISBN 978 1 4081 0140 7

### Note

While every effort has been made to ensure that the content of this book is as technically accurate and as sound as possible, neither the author nor the publishers can accept responsibility for any injury or loss sustained as a result of the use of this material.

A CIP catalogue record for this book is available from the British Library.

Cover photograph © Alamy
Illustrations by © Jeff Edwards

This book is produced using paper that is made from wood grown in managed, sustainable forests. It is natural, renewable and recyclable. The logging and manufacturing processes conform to the environmental regulations of the country of origin.

Typeset in Baskerville BE Regular by Palimpsest Book Production Limited, Grangemouth, Stirlingshire

Printed and bound at Graphycems in Spain.

# CONTENTS

# ACKNOWLEDGEMENTS

It is with great pleasure and with thanks to the team at A & C Black that I have the opportunity to revise and produce the 3rd edition of this, my first ever book in the Complete Guide series. The recent introduction of the New Fitness Instructing Level 3 qualifications, in the contexts of both Exercise to Music and also Exercise in Water (2007), has demanded a significant review of the original material to ensure it meets these additional requirements. This edition also includes chapter objectives and short answer revision questions to assist the learning process.

There are many people who I need to thank, for their support and encouragement:

- The late Lesley Mowbray of Central YMCA for whom I will always have great professional respect.
- My colleagues at Central YMCA Qualifications and YMCA Fitness Industry Training, with special thanks to Sheena Land (fellow aqua presenter) for contributing her 'Fish and Chips' choreography ideas.
- My partner Joe – for adding the tortoise (slower) approach to my hare (faster) approach to living!
- My mum, Mary Lawrence, for introducing me to exercise and activity and encouraging me to work in the fitness industry.
- Everyone who has ever participated in my land and water-based classes.
- Gaynor Curtis for her contribution of ideas for the deepwater section.
- The team at A & C Black for their positive encouragement and feedback regarding the writing of this 3rd edition.
- The Amateur Swimming Association (ASA) for promoting the book as part of their reading resources – thank you!

Happy aqua teaching to one and all!

# DEDICATION

I continue to dedicate the updated edition of this book to the memory of the late Lesley Mowbray – the founder of Central YMCA's Training and Development department, who sadly died of cancer at the age of 46 on 17th April 1998. Her vision, inspiration and dedication changed the face of exercise and fitness teaching in the UK. No individual has been more responsible for building the foundations for the standards relating to safe, effective exercise teaching than Lesley. May this book serve to preserve her in memory for all new instructors!

# INTRODUCTION

For centuries, water has provided a medium for the sport and recreation of different civilisations. It is well documented that the ancient Greeks and Romans used water for a variety of purposes. These included assisting with the alleviation of fatigue and low spirits, promoting cleanliness, and enhancing a general feeling of well-being.

In modern society, physiotherapists have for many years used water to assist with their treatments for the rehabilitation of injuries and other medical conditions. However, it is only more recently, approximately within the last three decades, that exercise and fitness professionals have adopted water as an alternative medium for delivering programmes to improve fitness and health. Indeed, there is currently a whole range of water-based exercise programmes available. These programmes attract a wide range of the population; people with different abilities and varying needs.

Exercising in water creates a totally different physical experience for the body than its land-based counterpart. This is because water has its own unique physical properties that will affect the body. These properties not only have an effect on the body systems, but also on how the body moves and the potential training benefits that can be obtained. It is neither safe nor effective to transfer our traditional land-based workouts directly into the water. Indeed, much thought needs to be given to the design of the water-based session and the exercises selected to achieve optimum benefits.

All instructors and enthusiasts using water as a training medium should have a sound basic knowledge of the following subject areas to assist with the design of safe and effective water-based training sessions:

1  Basic anatomy and physiology of the human body – exercise and fitness knowledge
2  The properties of water, their effects on the body and how they affect movement
3  Safe, effective exercises and session structure
4  Health and safety considerations for the pool environment
5  The ability, needs and requirements of the participants
6  Coaching strategies.

However, it is the application of this knowledge that is most important. The careful adaptation of exercises to utilise the properties of water will provide the first step towards structuring a safe and effective water-based training session. The needs of participants and environmental constraints should be identified and accommodated in the initial planning of the session. It is then up to the skills of the instructor to communicate to participants how to manipulate the water to gain optimum benefits.

The intention of this book is to provide a complete guide to exercise in water. It is assumed that the reader will have some basic knowledge of anatomy and physiology as applied to the exercising context. However, any technical terminology or concepts are explained as simply as possible and discussed in an applied sense throughout the book. This is to ensure that the book serves as an equally accessible and useful reference for the lay-person, as well as the fitness instructor. Those interested in training to teach water-based exercises should contact any of the training organisations listed at the back of this book, who offer training and assessment in a variety of exercise and fitness disciplines.

## How this book works

The book is divided into five main sections for ease of reference.

**Part 1** focuses on water, fitness and health. Chapter 1 explores the effects of the properties of water on the body. Chapter 2 explores the benefits of water-based exercise, and its potential contribution to the promotion of improved physical fitness and health for a wide variety of participants.

**Part 2** discusses the necessary considerations prior to planning a water-based exercise programme. Chapter 3 identifies the potential target groups and the information needed prior to their safe participation. Chapter 4 identifies the different pool environments and discusses how to adapt session content and structure for each one. It also explores further safety considerations related to the pool environment.

**Part 3** specifically looks at the structure and content of the water-based exercise programme. Chapter 5 identifies a range of different session formats. It also provides guidelines for an appropriate duration and intensity of a water-based programme for different populations. Chapters 6–11 explain and illustrate appropriate exercises for each component of the session and for different session formats. Chapter 12 provides ideas for using equipment and working in deeper water.

**Part 4** focuses on water-based training for specialist populations. Chapter 13 explains the benefits of water-based exercise for the sportsperson. Chapter 14 identifies the specialist considerations necessary for coaching seniors

in water. Chapter 15 explains how to adapt session structure ante- and post-natal. Persons wishing to train these populations should seek specialist training to equip them with the necessary knowledge and skills. YMCA Fitness Industry Training offers a range of training programmes to equip the teacher or instructor with the necessary knowledge and skills.

**Part 5** explores teaching using music and choreography. Chapter 16 explains appropriate teaching strategies for the exercise in water teacher. Chapter 17 discusses the use of music in a water-based exercise session, and choreography skills. Chapter 18 provides lesson plans for all components of the session, with and without equipment.

Ultimately, it should be recognised that, as the title of the book suggests, this is a complete guide to water-based exercise, which reflects the knowledge and experience of the author.

The content of this book is designed to reflect and meet some of the requirements for the Award Body Common Units in Exercise and Fitness Instruction (Exercise in Water) and provides some of the knowledge-base evidence (discussed in an applied Exercise in Water context) to meet the National Occupational Standards (NOS) in Fitness Instructing (Level 2 and 3). Many of the exercise and fitness topics discussed (energy systems, muscle and joint actions etc) are covered in greater detail in other specialist textbooks. A useful introductory text that also meets the requirements for the Level 2 and 3 Fitness Instructor qualifications is: *The Fitness Instructor's Handbook* by Morc Coulson also published by A&C Black (2007). A list of other recommended further reading and reference material is supplied at the end of the book. People interested in studying a specific knowledge area in greater depth should consider these references.

## Level 2 Instructing Exercise and Fitness

| Unit code | Unit Description |
| --- | --- |
| C35 | Deal with accidents and emergencies |
| D416 | Evaluate coaching sessions and deal with personal coaching practice |
| D417 | Support participants in developing and maintaining fitness |
| D414 | Plan and prepare a group water-based exercise session |
| D415 | Instruct a group water-based exercise session |

## Level 3 Instructing Exercise and Fitness

| Unit code | Unit Description |
| --- | --- |
| D437 | Deal with accidents and emergencies |
| D438 | Evaluate coaching sessions and deal with personal coaching practice |
| D439 | Support participants in developing and maintaining fitness |
| A318 | Plan and prepare a group water-based exercise session |
| D444 | Instruct a group water-based exercise session |

## Level 3 Core Exercise and Fitness Knowledge:

| | |
| --- | --- |
| 1 | Behaviour Change |
| 2 | Anatomy |
| 3 | Functional Kinesiology |
| 4 | Energy Systems |
| 5 | Concepts and Components of Fitness |

NB: Copies of the Award Body Common Units and National Occupational Standards can be obtained from the Sector Skills Council (Skills Active) and/or the Register of Exercise Professionals (REPs).

WATER AND FITNESS

**1**

# THE EFFECTS OF THE PHYSICAL PROPERTIES OF WATER

1

## OBJECTIVES

By the end of this chapter the reader will be able to:

- Describe the effects of buoyancy on the body
- Recognise how body composition will influence buoyancy and levels of flotation
- Recognise how body type may affect body composition and levels of buoyancy
- Recognise how distribution of body fat will affect flotation
- Recognise how air in the lungs may affect buoyancy
- Describe the different types of resistance (frontal, eddy and viscous) that will affect the body when exercising in water
- Describe how frontal resistance will affect muscle contraction in a water-based session
- Recognise how propulsive movements can be used to assist or resist movement when exercising in water
- Describe how propulsive movements can be used to maintain and regain balance
- Describe the effects of hydrostatic pressure on the body systems
- Recognise how water and air temperature will influence exercise selection and session structure.

## What is different about exercising in water?

When we exercise on dry land our skeletal, muscular, cardiovascular, respiratory and other body systems are greatly affected by the forces of gravity.

When we exercise in water the effects created by the gravitational pull on the body are reduced. However, water possesses its own unique properties which affect the body in a different way and provide us with a totally new experience. The deeper we submerge our bodies, the greater the effects of water and the lesser the effects of the gravitational pull.

A sound understanding of the properties of water and their effects on the body systems are essential for the instructor or enthusiast designing water-based exercise programmes. The effectiveness of any programme will ultimately be dependent on how well these properties are understood, and how well they are utilised to maximise the training benefits received. This chapter introduces the reader to buoyancy, resistance, temperature, hydrostatic pressure and their effects on the body. It also identifies and discusses the initial considerations when utilising the properties to optimise training benefits.

## What is buoyancy?

It is generally accepted that the theory of buoyancy was discovered by the Greek philosopher and mathematician Archimedes (287–212 BC). His theory suggests that when a body is immersed in water it will displace an amount of water equal to the mass of the body submerged. This displacement causes the water to rise and surround the body and will push it upwards and out towards the water surface.

## How does buoyancy affect the body?

Buoyancy creates the marvellous feeling of weightlessness and flotation that most of us experience when we are submerged in water.

When submerged in water to waist level the gravitational pull is reduced by 50 per cent. This means that we are partially affected by gravity and partially affected by buoyancy.

When submerged at chest depth the gravitational pull is reduced much further, approximately by 80 per cent. Therefore, the effects of gravity on our body are much lower and we are affected much more by buoyancy.

### NEED TO KNOW

When exercising in water the gravitational pull on the body is reduced according to the level of submersion. The body is, instead, affected by the buoyancy of the water. The deeper the body is submerged, the greater will be the effects of buoyancy.

The reduction of the gravitational pull and increased flotation provided by buoyancy will support our body frame. It will reduce the weight our joints are normally required to carry when standing or moving on land. This allows the joints to lift and separate and will decrease the compression they normally experience during land-based exercise programmes.

Most land-based exercise programmes involve the performance of some vigorous jogging and jumping activities that involve the body being lifted momentarily from the ground. These activities increase the weight borne by the joints, because the forces of gravity pull the bodyweight back down at a greater velocity, increasing the force exerted on the joints during landing. Exercise professionals traditionally classify such activities as high impact. A key disadvantage of these activities is that they place enormous stress on the joints and can therefore potentially increase the risk of injury. To enhance the safety of land-based training programmes the activities need to be altered to vary the impact and stress placed on the joints.

However, because the gravitational pull is reduced when immersed in water, the impact forces are lessened. Therefore, the impact normally received when performing such activities is dramatically reduced. They can therefore be performed for a longer duration and more frequently, without increasing the risk of injury. That is, of course, provided they are performed in an appropriate water depth by capable individuals.

The unique support that buoyancy provides to the skeletal system reduces the impact stress placed on the body during exercise. Therefore, water-based exercising can provide an excellent form of cross training for the sportsperson and exercise enthusiast alike. In addition, it provides the ideal medium for populations who need a more supportive environment, such as the injured or overweight.

Buoyancy will also naturally assist the flotation of our arms and legs (the body's levers) to the water surface. This can reduce the amount of muscle work necessary to maintain certain positions during exercise. For example, if standing on land with our arms stretched out to our sides in a crucifix position, our deltoid and upper portion of the trapezius muscle would need to contract statically (isometrically) to hold the position. This muscular contraction is necessary to overcome the force of gravity, which pulls the body and the body levers downwards. However, when our arms are submerged in water their weight is supported by the buoyancy, which pushes the body upwards. Therefore, these muscles will not need to work so hard, if at all, to hold the position. As a consequence, other movements of the arm can be performed with greater ease.

Buoyancy can therefore assist the performance of certain exercises. If it is utilised effectively in this way, it can promote the achievement of a greater range of motion in the moving joints, and improve mobility and flexibility. This is especially beneficial for participants with limited muscular strength and flexibility around their joints, who need extra support to perform such exercises. Buoyancy provides the support they need to move through a fuller range of motion.

However, buoyancy can also add resistance to movements. When pushing a body part down through the water there is a greater resistance for the muscles to overcome. This requires them to work harder and will therefore increase the intensity of the movement. If utilised effectively in this way, it will promote the improvement of muscular strength and endurance, which gives the body a toned appearance. The use of flotation equipment attached to the arms and legs will increase the effects of buoyancy, and further intensify the workload. The added flotation created by such devices provides an extra

resistance and requires greater effort from the muscles to overcome the buoyancy, and maintain balance. The use of flotation equipment is especially useful when designing programmes for fitter and stronger participants who need the extra resistance to challenge their muscles. However, less fit and specialist groups should use their body as a resistance and progress more steadily to using such devices.

## NEED TO KNOW

- Buoyancy changes the effects of the gravitational pull on the body.
- Buoyancy pushes the body upwards and out of the water.
- Buoyancy decreases the stress on weight-bearing joints and muscles.
- Working *with* buoyancy will assist with the improvement of mobility and flexibility.
- Working *against* buoyancy will assist with the improvement of local muscular strength and endurance, and muscle tone.

## What factors determine our level of buoyancy?

The degree to which a body will float is determined by three factors.

1 Body composition – the ratio of body fat to lean tissue (muscle and bone) carried by an individual.
2 The distribution of body fat, that is, where it is carried/deposited (for example, lower or upper body).
3 The air in the lungs.

# What factors affect body composition?

Our body composition is largely affected by our lifestyle and our eating habits. If we are inactive and eat too much then it is likely that we will have excess body fat. However, there are gender differences that will also affect our body composition. Women naturally tend to have and require higher proportions of body fat than men. In addition, we all inherit a genetic somatotype (body type). This may also have an effect on our body composition.

There are three main body types. These are illustrated below. Endomorphs, who tend to be shorter and rounder in appearance, carry a higher proportion of body fat. Ectomorphs, who tend to be taller and leaner in appearance, carry lower proportions of body fat and have a lower proportion of muscle. Mesomorphs, who tend to be more athletic in appearance, have broader shoulders, narrower hips and have greater muscularity. If our genetic parents are ectomorphic then it is more than likely we will inherit ectomorphic characteristics. Alternatively, if our parents are endomorphic, then it is more likely we will inherit endomorphic characteristics. However, it is common for us to possess characteristics of each of the different body types, although we will tend to have a bias towards one of these main types.

# How will having a muscular or leaner body type affect buoyancy?

Muscular (mesomorphic) or leaner (ectomorphic) body types are less buoyant. This is because they are composed of a higher proportion of leaner tissue such as muscle and bone, and a lower proportion of body fat. Muscle and bone have a greater density (are heavier) than

**Fig. 1.1** **Different body types (1) mesomorph; (2) endomorph; (3) ectomorph**

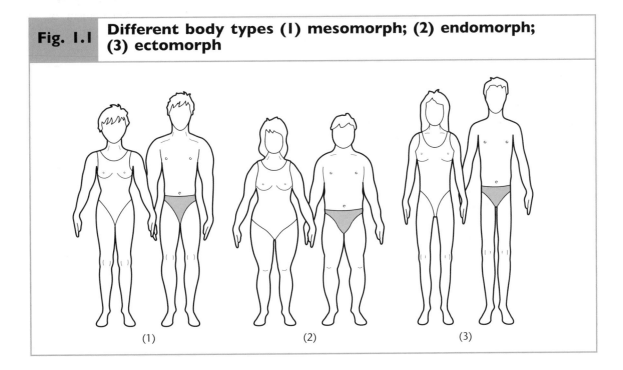

(1)    (2)    (3)

water, therefore they do not float so well and tend to sink. These body types are at an advantage when they need to move at a greater speed through the water. Their decreased ability to float and their smaller surface area (width and breadth) enables them to move more easily and at a faster pace. In addition, they tend to be more able to maintain a balanced position because of their more solid frame. They will therefore find it easier to perform exercises that require them to maintain a stationary position.

While leaner or muscular body types should exercise in chest depth water ideally to maximise the support buoyancy offers to their bones and joints, their joints will be under less stress if it is necessary for them to exercise in shallower water (waist depth). Leaner body types generally have a lower body weight, which reduces the load that the joints need to carry, providing less impact on their body. Muscular body types may be heavier, but generally have stronger muscles. Their strong muscular support will assist with the maintenance of correct joint alignment, keeping the joints in a stable position and reducing the stress placed on them.

When exercising in very deep water (2m/6ft) these body types will probably need the assistance of a buoyancy aid to assist flotation. Without it, they will spend much of their workout expending energy to maintain flotation, not on the performance of the specific exercise.

## How will having a less lean (higher body fat ratio) body type affect buoyancy?

Rounder (endomorphic) and curvaceous body types are more buoyant. This is because they are composed of a higher proportion of body fat and a lower proportion of lean tissue. They float much more easily than their leaner colleagues because body fat has a lower density (is lighter) than water. Their increased flotation and buoyancy makes it harder for these body types to move quickly in the water. This is because they frequently have a larger surface area (width and breadth) to drag through the water. This requires them to work harder and exert a greater force to create movement.

Additionally, their increased flotation makes it harder for them to balance and maintain a stable position. Therefore, when performing exercises that create a lot of turbulence (movement) in the water, it may be necessary for them to exercise in a shallower depth of water to maintain a stationary position and to avoid being thrown off balance and dragged off by the water. However, if such adaptations are necessary, it must be recognised that exercising in shallower water will increase the gravitational pull on their body. Therefore, if the activity requires jumping or jogging movements, greater stress will be placed on their joints. This is because the mass of their body adds greater weight for their joints to carry and, in many instances, the lack of strong muscular support reduces their ability to maintain correct alignment. Exercises in shallower water may therefore require further adaptation to promote safer performance. Ultimately, exercising in chest depth water is far less stressful and more supportive for these body types.

When exercising in very deep water these body types have an advantage, since normally they do not need to expend so much energy trying to maintain flotation. They can often therefore exercise more comfortably and for a longer duration than their leaner colleagues without the use of a buoyancy aid. This is of course dependent on the fitness level of the individual and their confidence in water.

# How will distribution of body fat affect buoyancy and flotation?

An individual's flotation is also determined by where they store and carry the majority of their body fat. Some individuals have a greater proportion of their body fat distributed in the lower body, giving them a pear-shaped appearance – generally women. Alternatively, other individuals have a greater proportion of their body fat distributed in the upper body, giving them an apple-shaped appearance – generally men. When the fat is stored in the lower body, the legs and hips tend to be more buoyant. They will therefore float in a more horizontal position (*see* Fig. 1.2(a) below). However, when the fat is stored around the upper body, the trunk will be more buoyant and flotation will be in a more vertical position (*see* Fig. 1.2(b), page 8).

## NEED TO KNOW

Summary of the effects of body composition on buoyancy
- Muscular and leaner body types are less buoyant, more stable, and can move more quickly through water.
- Fatter body types are more buoyant, less stable, and cannot move so quickly through water.
- Leaner and muscular body types are under less stress than fatter body types when exercising in shallower water; they cannot maintain flotation so economically in deeper water.
- Fatter body types are able to maintain flotation more effectively than leaner or muscular body types when exercising in deeper water. However, their joints are under greater stress during shallow water activities.

## Fig. 1.2a  Distribution of body fat

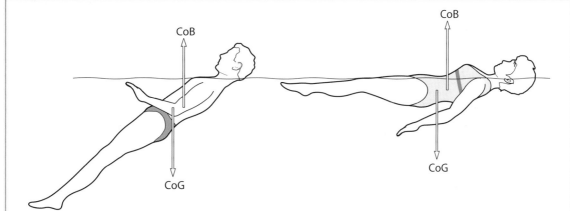

Note: Centre of buoyancy (CoB) and Centre of gravity (CoG). The centre of buoyancy is slightly lower when body fat is distributed around the lower body. It is higher when the body fat is distributed around the upper body

| Fig. 1.2b | Distribution of body fat |
| --- | --- |

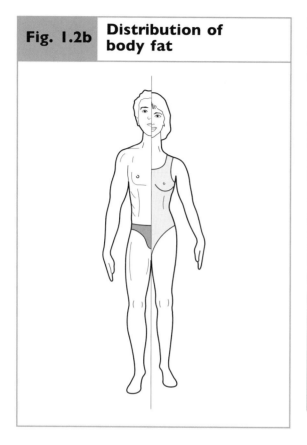

have greater rest between bouts of the same activity (sets) in the same exercise programme. The different positions in which to perform activities at the poolside are illustrated in Fig. 1.3 on page 9.

### NEED TO KNOW

Summary of the effects of distribution of body fat

- If fat is stored in the upper body (apple shape) the legs will tend to sink, making it difficult to maintain flotation of the legs during exercises that demand the legs to float upwards.
- If fat is stored in the lower body (pear shape) the legs will tend to float, making it more difficult to maintain a more vertical alignment.
- Alternative positions need to be offered to accommodate different levels of flotation.

The distribution of body fat and position of flotation is very important when designing exercises. It requires a range of alternative positions to be considered and offered to allow participants to perform exercises comfortably. Exercises that require the lower body to maintain a horizontal position will be uncomfortable for those with muscular legs. They will exert more effort trying to maintain the flotation of the legs, rather than performing the exercise. It is therefore advisable to provide them with exercises that position the body vertically. However, naturally horizontal floaters have more difficulty maintaining a vertical position. They need greater fixation of their abdominal muscles to perform exercises safely. This may require them to perform a lower number of repetitions and

## How will air in lungs affect buoyancy/flotation?

The greater the volume of air in the lungs, for example during inhalation, the higher the body will float in the water; the less air there is in the lungs, for example during exhalation, the lower it will float. This can be experienced by performing a mushroom float in water before and after exhalation (*see* Fig. 1.4 on page 10). This is perhaps a less significant factor during water-based exercise. However, it is useful for determining a person's level of buoyancy and the flotation they are likely to experience. It is not an appropriate method for determining the flotation of non-swimmers or those less confident in water.

| Fig. 1.3 | **Different positions in which to perform exercises at the poolside** |
| --- | --- |

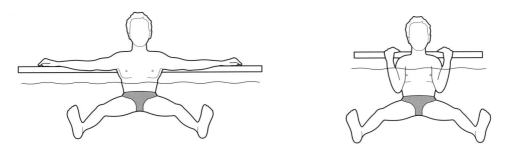

Note: The arm position can be altered in both positions to suit individual requirements.

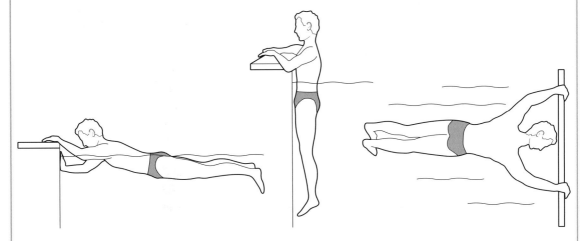

Note: A variety of arm grips and lying positions should be offered to accommodate all body types. This will ensure individuals are comfortable in the exercise, and should improve their performance.

## NEED TO KNOW

- Air in the lungs will affect flotation.
- When there is less air in lungs (exhalation) the body will sink.
- When there is more air in the lungs (inhalation) the body will float.

| Fig. 1.4 | **Level of flotation determined by air in the lungs** |
| --- | --- |

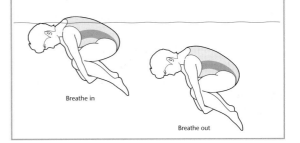

Breathe in

Breathe out

## How will the resistance of water affect the body?

There are three types of resistance created by the water. These are frontal resistance, eddy resistance or eddy drag, and viscous resistance. Each of these has a different effect on the body, and will therefore be discussed individually. However, one should recognise that when moving in water they will each be acting on the body simultaneously.

## What is frontal resistance?

When the body is immersed in water it is surrounded by a medium that exerts a constant and multi-dimensional resistance to its every movement. This resistance is approximately 12 times more resistant than air and requires the body to work three times harder than when exercising on dry land. Every movement potentially demands a greater muscular exertion and greater energy expenditure to overcome the resistance. Therefore, if this resistance is utilised effectively it can create the necessary overload for the muscular and cardiovascular systems that will induce the desired training effects. It can also be utilised to promote the burning of calories that potentially assist with the control and management of body weight.

### NEED TO KNOW

- Water provides a resistance to movement that is approximately 12 times greater than the resistance of air.

## How will frontal resistance affect movement?

The resistance water provides to movement will reduce the speed at which the body can move. All movements in water will need to be performed at approximately half the speed that they are performed on land, although the speed may need to be reduced further for more buoyant body types or for people exercising in deeper water, due to the extra resistance provided to their movement. Additionally, all movements in water will need to maximise the use of the body's levers through a larger range of motion. This will increase the surface area being moved, which adds resistance and therefore promotes a greater effect.

However, it should be recognised that if movements are too slow, and through too large a range of motion, they may be of no benefit at all. This is because buoyancy and flotation will be assisting the movement of the body. Alternatively, if movements are too quick and utilise too small a range of motion then they will be equally ineffective. This is because they will not maximise the drag of a body part or its surface area appropriately through the water, reducing the muscular effort required to work effectively. Figs 1.5, 1.6 and 1.7 illustrate how the intensity of movements can be heightened by increasing the surface area moved through the water.

Ultimately, the speed of movement in water will need to be slower for all participants. However, a combination of relatively moderate pace, full range of motion activities, and slightly faster, smaller range of motion activities, creates an effective mode of training. This is of course dependent on the body type and fitness levels of participants, and the depth of water they are exercising in. When working with less fit groups the use of a smaller surface area, shorter leverage

| Fig. 1.5 | Surface area of arm leverage to increase resistance (1 = easiest; 5 = hardest) |
|---|---|

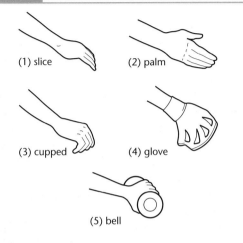

(1) slice  (2) palm

(3) cupped  (4) glove

(5) bell

Note: Increase the intensity of the movement by adding greater surface area to the lever. Reduce surface area to allow for greater speed of movement. Using equipment will also add to the surface area moved through the water.

and slower pace movements may well be sufficient for them to obtain the desired training benefits. Alternatively, working with fitter groups may require the more regular use of slightly faster moves with longer leverage and a greater surface area to work at an appropriate intensity. Fitter participants may also need to exercise using flotation equipment, which increases buoyancy, adds resistance to movement, and demands greater muscular and cardiovascular effort.

However, the effectiveness of all water-based movements will also be determined by the force exerted by the body part(s) being moved. The greater the force exerted, the greater will be the effort. It is therefore essential that exercisers are encouraged to work the water to maximise the gains they receive. Pulling, kicking or pushing the water to the best of their ability are essential instructions to maximise the benefits received.

| Fig. 1.6 | Surface area of the body adding resistance to movement |
|---|---|

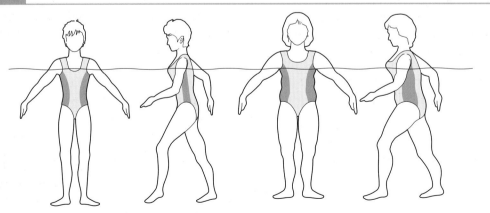

Note: The larger body frame will not be able to move so quickly through the water in any direction. This is due to a naturally greater surface area that needs to be dragged through the water.

## Fig. 1.7 Extending the lever increases the resistance and so is harder work

Shorter lever            Longer lever

Note: Movements using shorter levers can be performed more quickly than movements using longer levers.

## How will frontal resistance affect muscle contraction?

The resistance to movements in all directions will also alter the way in which the muscles contract. On dry land our muscles are working and contracting constantly to overcome the forces of gravity, which pull us down. In water, the amount of work required from our muscles to support our bodyweight is reduced. This is due to the buoyancy of water, which causes us to float. However, our muscles are still working and contracting to maintain balance and prevent excessive movement which is created by our flotation.

When we are moving or lifting a resistance on land, our muscles have to contract to overcome the forces of gravity. As we lift the weight of our body or an external resistance such as a hand weight upwards, our muscles will contract and get shorter (concentric muscle work). Lowering our bodyweight or the external resistance will require our muscles to contract and get longer (eccentric muscle work).

For example, lifting the leg to a horizontal position (hip flexion) will require the hip flexor muscles (iliopsoas and rectus femoris) to contract concentrically. Lowering the leg back to the floor (hip extension) will require the same muscles to contract eccentrically.

### NEED TO KNOW

On land:
- Movements that lift the body and/or levers upwards against the force of gravity will bring about concentric muscle work. The muscles shorten to bring about the movement.
- Movements that lower the body and/or levers back down to the start position will bring about eccentric muscle work. The muscles lengthen to lower the body down with the force of gravity.

When we move in water, our body has a different resistance to overcome. The majority of muscular contractions are concentric due to the resistance to movement in all directions. For example, when the arms are outstretched to the sides of the body and push forward through the water, the muscles of the chest (pectorals) will contract and get shorter (concentric muscle work), and when the arms are moved back, the opposite muscles (trapezius and rhomboids) will also contract and get shorter (concentric muscle work). All movements working across the resistance of the water will demand this 'dual-concentric' muscle work (*see* Fig. 1.8).

An advantage of these dual-concentric muscular contractions is that a larger proportion of skeletal muscles are required to work. This can assist with the development of a more balanced muscular workout, and potentially promote greater improvements in postural alignment. Additionally, the reduction in the amount of eccentric work can eliminate the muscle soreness normally experienced a few days after exercising on dry land. This is because unfamiliar eccentric muscle work is that which is most likely to cause this soreness. Knowing that aches and pains will be minimal should enhance the appeal of water-based exercise for many of the population. Those who still feel that without the pain there will be no gain need to be re-educated. Firstly, they should recognise that pain is not necessary to achieve an effective workout. Secondly, they should appreciate that the supportive properties of water will naturally decrease the stress on the body. Finally, they should recognise that the added resistance to movement in all directions gives great potential to challenge the muscles quite sufficiently.

If flotation equipment is used, then muscle contractions may alter. The dual-concentric muscle work will be maintained while working across the water, but will change when working against buoyancy. For example, an elbow curl on dry land will require the biceps muscle to contract concentrically to lift the weight up and eccentrically to lower the weight back down. In water, the triceps muscle will contract concentrically to press the water bell down through the water and eccentrically to return the water bell to the water's surface (*see* Fig. 1.9). Muscle contraction appears then to work in reverse to how it works on land: upside down and reverse kinesiology. However, the contraction of muscles during water-based exercise programmes is an area where much further research is required. The type of contraction that occurs will be affected by individual buoyancy/flotation, the specific exercise being performed, and the amount of force exerted by the individual performing the exercise.

**Fig. 1.8** **Muscular contraction of the pectorals and trapezius when horizontally flexing and extending the shoulder in water**

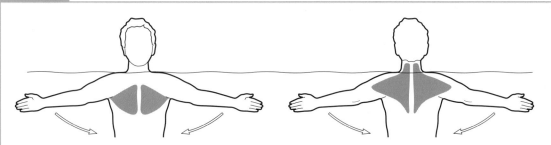

Note: The pectorals contract concentrically to pull the arms forwards through the water. The trapezius and rhomboids contract concentrically to pull the arms backwards through the water.

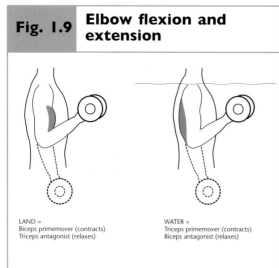

**Fig. 1.9** **Elbow flexion and extension**

LAND =
Biceps primemover (contracts)
Triceps antagonist (relaxes)

WATER =
Triceps primemover (contracts)
Biceps antagonist (relaxes)

Note: On land the biceps contract concentrically to lift the weight and eccentrically to lower it. In water the triceps muscle contracts concentrically to press the water bell down, and eccentrically to return it to the surface.

## What is eddy resistance?

Eddy resistance or turbulence is created when a body or a body part moves through the water. When a greater number of body parts are required to move, the eddy resistance and turbulence is increased. Travelling movements, in particular, appear to increase the formation of eddy currents and create greater turbulence. In addition, the water will become more turbulent and more eddy currents will be formed when movements are performed at a greater speed, and when the force exerted by the body or body part is stronger. Needless to say, these forces are increased further when a larger number of bodies are moving or exercising in the water at the same time. When participants are placed in random positions around the pool, and are moving in different ways, the eddy

currents appear to be slightly greater. When participants are organised and encouraged to move in a more linear and streamlined fashion, the eddy currents appear to be slightly lower. Ultimately, the greater the level of turbulence created, the greater will be the resistance to movement.

>
> **NEED TO KNOW**
>
> Eddy resistance will be greater when:
> - The exercise speed is faster.
> - There are lots of travelling movements in different directions.
> - There are more people working in the pool.
> - The poolside is higher than the water's edge, and the water hits against the pool wall.

## How does eddy resistance affect movement?

Turbulence (eddy currents) adds further resistance to the body movements, making it harder for the body to move and maintain balance. It requires the strong fixation of the abdominal muscles, and equally strong propulsive movements, to maintain balance and create further movement. In particular, it will restrict and reduce the speed at which changes of direction and changes of movement can be executed safely while using the correct technique.

While quick changes of direction can increase the intensity of the workout, they should only be performed by people with sufficient strength to fixate the abdominals and perform the powerful propulsive movements that need to occur to maintain balance and achieve movement in the opposite direction. If working with groups of a lower fitness level, the use of stationary movements between bouts of travel can decrease the intensity. This will allow time for the eddy currents to subside, and for the body to regain its balance, decreasing the power of the propulsive movement necessary to create travel. Additionally, since more buoyant body types are less able to maintain balance, they should be advised to exercise in shallower water or on the outside of the group if quick direction changes are required.

## What is viscous resistance?

All fluids or liquids have a viscosity or thickness of flow. The greater the viscosity, the greater will be the resistance to movement. Oil is a liquid, which naturally has a greater viscosity than water, therefore it exerts a greater resistance, making it harder to move an object through oil than to move an object through water. For example, if stirring oil and water with a spoon, the spoon will move more quickly and easily through the water. However, as the temperature of any liquid increases, so the viscosity decreases. Therefore, when a liquid is warmed, it will flow more freely and provide less resistance to movement.

## How does viscous resistance affect movement?

The viscosity of the water is also affected by its temperature and the temperature of the surrounding air. The colder the water, and the colder the surrounding air, the greater will be its viscosity and resistance to movement. As air temperature and water temperature increase, the viscosity of water will decrease, thus providing less resistance to movement. This has

less of an effect on water-based exercise programmes, since such programmes are normally performed in warmer water temperatures that allow the body to move more quickly. However, a long-distance swimmer will potentially achieve a faster time if they swim when the weather and subsequent water temperatures are warmer and the water is less viscous.

### NEED TO KNOW

**Summary of the effects of resistance**

- The frontal and viscous resistance of water will require greater effort from our muscles to create movement.
- Frontal resistance will require predominantly concentric muscle contractions to create movement. This potentially provides a more balanced muscular workout.
- Eddy resistance makes it harder to change direction quickly and requires greater muscular effort to maintain balance and to overcome this resistance.
- Eddy resistance offers a challenge to core stability.
- Larger body frames have a greater surface area to drag through water, which adds further resistance and intensity to their movements.
- Leaner or muscular body types may require the use of flotation equipment to increase the resistance provided to their movement.

## What are propulsive movements?

Propulsive movements are the movements of our body levers (the arms and legs) which are necessary to overcome and manipulate the resistant properties of water.

---

### NEED TO KNOW

Propulsive movements can be used to:
- initiate or create travel in a desired direction
- maintain a balanced and/or stationary position during activity
- maintain flotation during deep water activities
- regain an upright position when balance is lost.

---

Swimmers move with relative ease and confidence in water; they therefore tend to perform the necessary propulsive movements fairly naturally. Alternatively, non-swimmers and those less confident in water appear to move less comfortably in water. They tend to be less familiar and less skilled at performing the propulsive movements that are necessary to manipulate the water in the appropriate way. It is therefore essential that they are coached and encouraged to develop these skills. Indeed, learning how to manipulate the water may increase their confidence in water and encourage them to learn to swim. This can provide them with yet another form of water activity to enjoy.

Propulsive movements can be used to assist or resist movement. They can assist and improve the performance of specific exercises by all participants. Alternatively, they can resist movement and, if necessary, can provide a way of creating further challenges for fitter participants. Providing they are coached effectively, they will maximise the effectiveness of the water-based exercise programme.

Sir Isaac Newton defined three laws of motion. Each contributes in some way to the movement of the body during water-based activity. However, the third law is that which affects almost every water-based movement. This law states that for every action there is an equal and opposite reaction.

## How can propulsive movements be used to initiate or create movement?

When the water is pushed or pulled in a specific direction (action) by one or more of the body levers, the body will travel in the opposite direction (reaction). The action and reaction created in kicking, pushing or pulling the water in a specific direction is outlined in table 1.1 opposite. The longer the lever initiating the movement and the stronger the force exerted by the muscles moving the lever, the greater will be the travel one experiences. Travelling movements in water are those that are more intense, due to the movement of the centre of buoyancy through the water. These movements can therefore be manipulated to create the desired intensity for the water-based exercise session.

| Table 1.1 | The action and reaction created by kicking, pushing or pulling the water in a specific direction | |
|---|---|---|
| **Action** | | **Reaction** |
| Pushing, pulling or kicking the water forwards | | The body will travel backwards |
| Pushing, pulling or kicking the water backwards | | The body will travel forwards |
| Pushing, pulling or kicking the water to the right side | | The body will travel to the left |
| Pushing, pulling or kicking the water to the left side | | The body will travel to the right |

Note: A longer lever exerting a stronger force (action) will create greater movement or travel in the opposite direction (reaction), than a shorter lever exerting less force.

| Fig. 1.10a | Synergistic or opposing muscle movement while jogging in water |
|---|---|

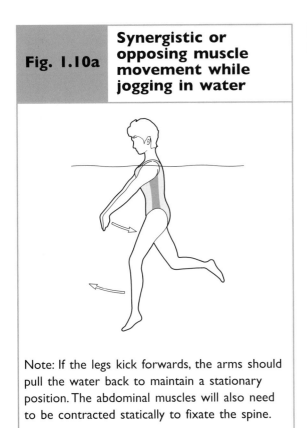

Note: If the legs kick forwards, the arms should pull the water back to maintain a stationary position. The abdominal muscles will also need to be contracted statically to fixate the spine.

| Fig. 1.10b | Synergistic or opposing muscle movement of the arm while performing a lateral leg raise |
|---|---|

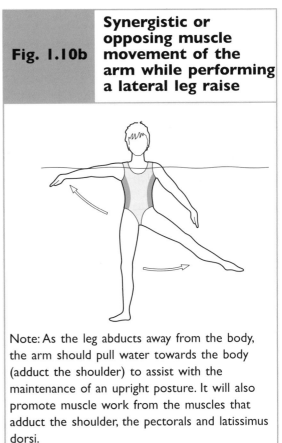

Note: As the leg abducts away from the body, the arm should pull water towards the body (adduct the shoulder) to assist with the maintenance of an upright posture. It will also promote muscle work from the muscles that adduct the shoulder, the pectorals and latissimus dorsi.

## How can propulsive movements be used to maintain balance and a stationary exercising position?

Movement of a body lever will create a movement in the opposite direction. Therefore, strong fixation of the abdominal muscles will be necessary to assist with the maintenance of balance and prevent unwanted movement in the opposite direction. An equally strong opposing or synergistic propulsive movement from another body part will provide further assistance to the maintenance of a stationary position (*see* Figs 1.10(a) and (b)). The opposing propulsive movement will counteract the forces of the primary action and, providing the forces exerted by the two body parts are equal, then the body should remain in the same position throughout the performance of the exercise.

Participants with leaner and less buoyant body types may be able to balance effectively without the use of opposing movements. They may well be able to maintain stability quite naturally while performing the lateral leg raise (*see* Fig. 1.10(b)). Positioning them in deeper water will make this harder for them. Additionally, if they kick the water forwards (*see* Fig. 1.10(a)) they may still be able to travel forwards when using an opposing propulsive movement of the arm. This is because their leaner frame (smaller surface area) makes it easier for them to move through water. Once again, increasing the depth in which they exercise will make this harder. Needless to say this should only be encouraged for those confident in water.

When performing upper body exercises in the centre of the pool it is advisable to offer the option of two basic leg stances (*see* Fig. 1.11). Participants should be allowed to select the one that allows them to maintain a balanced posture throughout the performance of the exercise.

The position they favour may be determined by the strength of their abdominal muscles, the depth of water and their body type. Participants with weaker abdominal muscles, and/or more buoyant body types, should be offered the alternative of exercising in shallower water to assist balance. Alternatively, the exercise may need to be adapted slightly so they can use the poolside or a flotation device to assist their stability and performance of the exercise.

The performance of lower body exercises in the centre of the pool can be assisted by the opposing movement of both arms. This will assist the maintenance of balance and an upright posture. Fig. 1.10(b) on page 17 illustrates this action using one arm to assist balance. Alternatively, a sculling movement of the arms can be used. Sculling movements are particularly useful to assist balance during the performance of static stretches in the middle of the pool.

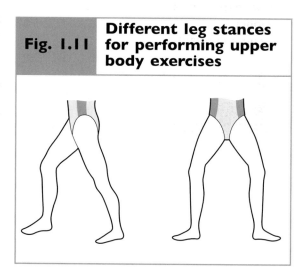

**Fig. 1.11 Different leg stances for performing upper body exercises**

## What is sculling?

Sculling is an oscillating movement of the arm and hand. Synchronised swimmers use a variety of skilled sculling techniques to assist with their performance of choreographed movement routines in water. It is not necessary for the general exerciser to perform such advanced sculling techniques. However, a version of such techniques can be used by exercisers to assist balance when exercising in the centre of the pool (*see* Fig. 1.12). This basic form of sculling involves positioning the hand with the little finger tilting upwards and rotating the arm in a figure-of-eight motion with the wrist leading the movement.

## Coaching points for sculling

- Keep arms under the water, with elbows straight.
- If both hands are used, keep them at the same depth.
- Hands should be slightly cupped with fingers extended.
- Rotate from the shoulders in a figure-of-eight motion.
- Keep a constant rhythm.

| Fig. 1.12 | **Sculling to assist balance during the performance of a quadriceps stretch** |
|---|---|

## How can propulsive movements be used to assist flotation in deeper water?

Fatter body types are more buoyant. Therefore, they will find it easier to maintain flotation in deeper water. However, all body types need some assistance to maintain their flotation. The key issue is the amount of energy they expend doing so. To keep the body up to the surface and out of the water will require the water to be pushed downwards in the opposite direction to which the body wants to move. This can be achieved by using a sculling movement of the arm, where the position of the hand is flatter and the arm is oscillated to push the water down. Alternatively, it can be achieved by treading water with the legs (*see* Fig. 1.13).

| Fig. 1.13 | **Treading water with the feet pushing down** |
|---|---|

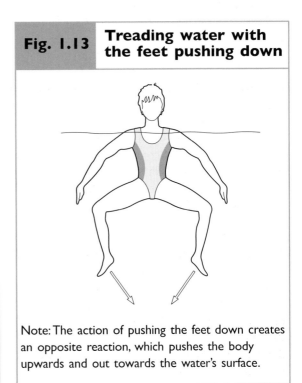

Note: The action of pushing the feet down creates an opposite reaction, which pushes the body upwards and out towards the water's surface.

## How can propulsive movements be used to regain balance?

A participant's ability to maintain balance in water is affected by the buoyancy of their body type and their skills at manipulating the water. Non-swimmers and those less confident in water are less skilled at manipulating the water and are therefore potentially those most likely to be thrown off balance during water-based activities. Losing the security of having their feet positioned on the pool floor can be a terrifying experience for those who are not confident in water. It will probably cause them to panic and move the water in a way which hinders their return to a vertical position. It is therefore essential that they are coached to develop the skills necessary to regain an upright and balanced position. Indeed, this is perhaps the most useful aid to performance an instructor can provide. It allows participants to feel more secure and proficient at keeping themselves safe.

The skills required to regain a vertical stance when the body loses balance in water use the principles of action and reaction. If the body slips and falls forwards or backwards in the water, the water needs to be pulled down (action) and the knees tucked up and under the body to regain balance in an upward position (the desired reaction – *see* Fig. 1.14). If participants are not able to perform these skills they should be advised to exercise in shallower water and closer to the poolside. The lifeguard should also be notified of their position. Proficiency of these skills is also essential prior to the performance of deep-water exercises or exercises using flotation devices that attach to the ankles (see fig. 1.14 opposite).

## What is hydrostatic pressure?

Water exerts a pressure on the whole body as it becomes immersed in water. The pressure exerted is proportional to the depth at which the body is immersed. Therefore, the deeper the body is submerged the greater will be the pressure applied by the water.

This pressure creates a feeling of tightness around the body, rather like the pressure of a bandage. It is this pressure that leaves our muscles feeling relaxed and our body lighter and refreshed after being immersed in water.

However, the pressure exerted on the thorax may create tightness in the chest area, making us more conscious of our breathing. This may create discomfort for some participants, particularly asthmatics. It is therefore advisable that they exercise in shallower water to avoid any discomfort created if they experience difficulties when breathing.

## How does hydrostatic pressure affect our body?

Hydrostatic pressure improves the circulation of blood around the body. Therefore, during water-based exercising the blood is distributed more evenly. Alternatively, land-based exercise programmes require the blood to be re-distributed to the working muscles. Specifically, the supply of blood to the kidneys is reduced and diverted to the muscles where it is most needed. However, because the circulation of blood is improved, this re-distribution of blood is unnecessary during water-based activities. Therefore, the kidneys are more active. This is why participants frequently need to leave the pool and go to the toilet during water-based activity. This is advantageous for those retaining excess fluid: they will be able to urinate more

**Fig. 1.14** **Regaining balance after a forward (top) or backward (bottom) fall in the water**

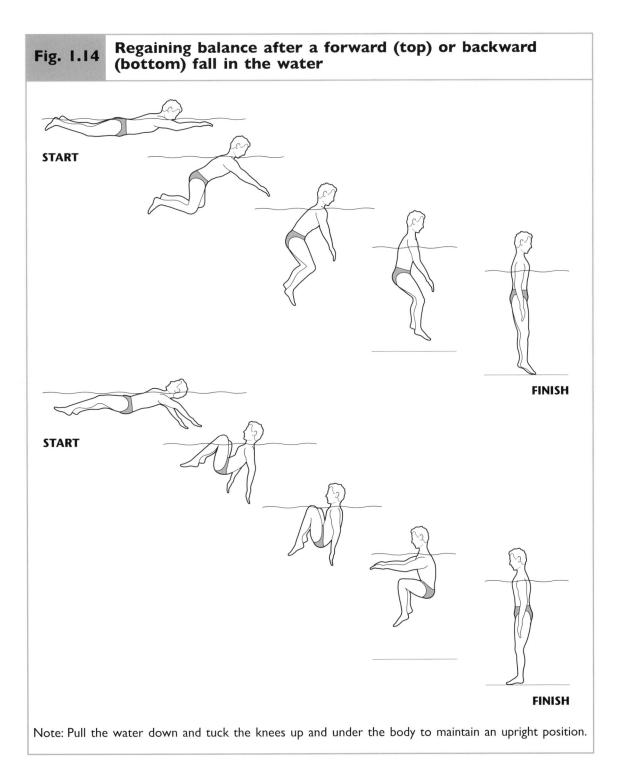

START

FINISH

START

FINISH

Note: Pull the water down and tuck the knees up and under the body to maintain an upright position.

readily, which may assist with the removal of some of the excess fluid they are carrying.

The pressure exerted on our body by the water will also promote the circulation of a greater volume of blood through the heart and vascular systems. This potentially increases the amount of blood pumped around the body in each contraction of the heart (stroke volume), and the amount of blood that travels through the heart each minute (cardiac output). This improvement to the circulation of blood may contribute to the lower working heart rate frequently reported by participants during water-based exercise. This infers that the heart is potentially placed under less stress during water-based activities, since it does not have to work so hard to pump the blood around the body. However, it raises a safety issue that needs to be considered when dealing with rehabilitated cardiac patients. This is whether their hearts would be able to cope with the increase of blood flow. Indeed, the level of intensity and possibly the depth of immersion would need to be reduced dramatically to maximise the safety of their workout. It is strongly advised that such participants are only accepted and coached by people who have undertaken specialist training to deal with their requirements (ideally physiotherapists); and only after approval from their doctor.

This pressure will also encourage a more effective return of venous blood back to the heart. This decreases the risk of blood pooling in the lower extremities and will potentially place less stress on the valves, which prevent back flow of blood in the veins. This is advantageous for those with varicose veins and makes water-based exercising a most suitable medium to improve their fitness. In addition, the reduced risk of blood pooling will allow participants to lower the intensity of their movements in water at a slightly faster rate than they are safely able to do on land. The improved venous return will prevent them experiencing dizziness or fainting, which is likely to occur if they stop too quickly during land-based exercise programmes. The improvement of the circulation of blood may also potentially contribute to the more effective removal of lactic acid to the liver. It could be hypothesised that this, and the increase of blood and oxygen through the body tissues, promotes greater use of the aerobic energy system to fuel activities. Indeed, water-based exercising is generally more comfortable and there is less likelihood of experiencing muscle soreness during or after the water-based workout.

There are additional benefits to be gained by those recovering from injury. The pressure of the water forces fluid from the cells of the injured body part into the capillaries (small blood vessels) and into the circulatory system. This can help to decrease the swelling in the injured area and, in turn, may reduce the pain experienced. It is frequently the excess of fluid that presses on nerve-endings and causes this pain. The effects of hydrostatic pressure, combined with the support provided by buoyancy, makes water an ideal medium for the treatment and rehabilitation of injuries. However, once again it is essential that referral from a doctor is obtained and the instructor is qualified and equipped to deal with the special requirements.

## NEED TO KNOW

Summary of the effects of hydro-static pressure

- Improves the circulation of blood through the kidneys, promoting urination and decreasing the retention of excess fluid.
- Improves the circulation of blood through the heart, which contributes to a lower heart rate during exercise, and effective delivery of oxygen to the muscles.
- Improves the circulation of venous blood, decreasing stress on the valves and reducing the risk of blood pooling.
- Improves the circulation of blood through the muscles and assists with the removal of lactic acid to the liver.
- Provides a massaging effect to the body, which can reduce muscle tension and leave the body feeling less stressed.

# How do we lose heat from the body?

The normal body temperature is approximately 37°C (98.6°F). This is to some extent variable throughout the day. However, we are normally able to maintain a constant temperature either through movement, the addition of extra clothing, or shivering. There are different ways in which we lose heat: by convection, conduction and evaporation.

## Convection

This occurs when the body comes into contact with air or water that is of a lower temperature than its own. The air or water is warmed by its contact with the body and then carried away. Thus, the body temperature is reduced and the body becomes cooler.

## Conduction

This is the transference of heat away from the body by the substance with which it is in contact. Water conducts heat more effectively than air, which is why it has a greater cooling effect on our body.

## Evaporation

The third way that we can lose heat is through perspiration or sweating, that is, the evaporation of water from the skin. This is the main way in which we maintain an appropriate temperature and prevent ourselves from overheating during dry land activities. However, in water we perspire very little, if at all. Only the body parts not immersed in water will lose heat by perspiring. Fortunately, water assists with our cooling and the maintenance of an appropriate body temperature. However, if the pool temperature is too low it may cool us down too much, or, if it is too hot, we may not cool off sufficiently, causing us to dehydrate and overheat.

# How does water temperature affect the body?

Immersion in water generally has a cooling effect on the body. Some participants see this as an advantage since they will not be hot and sweaty throughout the workout. However, this may also create the misconception that they are exercising at a lower intensity. Additionally, the body will cool down approximately four times quicker than in air. This may leave participants feeling cold, unless sufficient activities are included to maintain a comfortable body temperature. The rate at which the body will lose heat is determined by the actual temperature of the water, the air temperature of the surrounding environment, and the amount of natural insulation provided by body fat and muscle.

Initial immersion into cooler water temperatures will cause the surface blood vessels to constrict. This is because the blood will temporarily be diverted away from the skin to the central organs to maintain their core temperature. This vaso-constriction may create an initial increase in heart rate and blood pressure. However, when the body becomes acclimatised to its new environment and warming activities start to occur, the blood vessels will once again dilate and the blood pressure and heart rate will normalise. Exercising in water that is too cool may maintain this vaso-constriction. This will increase the energy we expend via shivering to maintain a comfortable body temperature. It may also reduce the transportation and consumption of oxygen, which is essential for optimal training benefits to be received. Alternatively, exercising in a pool that is too hot may cause us to overheat and potentially dehydrate. A key disadvantage of not sweating is that we are unable to cool ourselves effectively when working in very hot pools.

When exercising in pools where the air temperature is lower than that of the water, the body will cool more rapidly. This is more frequently the case in larger swimming pools where one or more of the walls leads directly to the outside of the building, and are less effectively insulated. Smaller pools that are positioned in the centre of a building and surrounded by other rooms tend to be more effectively insulated and have higher air temperatures. If the air temperature is higher than the pool temperature, the body will stay warmer, making it more comfortable for participants. However, the instructor may experience dehydration and overheat a lot quicker when working on the poolside. They should therefore replenish the fluid lost by drinking water more frequently, and splashing themselves with water to stay cooler.

Ultimately, the temperature of the water should not be below 29°C (84°F) and the surrounding air temperature should be slightly higher, although some may argue that this pool temperature is too low. In addition, it should not exceed 32°C (90°F). The suitability of the pool temperature is dependent on the level of intensity of the activities being performed and the requirements of the group performing them. A less active or less energetic session may be safe to perform in a hotter pool. Reasonably well-insulated body types may be comfortable performing a more active session in a cooler pool.

## How will body composition affect maintenance of body temperature?

Ectomorphic body types are leaner and have less subcutaneous fat and less muscle mass. They will therefore be more susceptible to the cooling effects of water than the other body types. Mesomorphic body types are to some extent insulated by their muscular tissue and can therefore maintain a more comfortable body temperature for longer. Endomorphic body types have a greater covering of body fat which acts as an insulator against the cold. However, this insulation can cause them to overheat if working too intensely and in pools that are very warm.

## How can we tell if participants are sufficiently warm?

The most effective way of discovering whether participants are warm enough is to ask them at regular intervals throughout the session. If they respond negatively at any time, the intensity of the activity can be increased slightly to maintain a comfortable temperature. Alternatively, the visual signs that indicate whether they are becoming too cold are pinched facial expressions and hunched shoulders. In addition, the appearance of goosebumps, which are caused by the contraction of the erector pilae muscles that extend the hairs on the body in an attempt to maintain warmth, is a sure sign of an uncomfortable temperature. Further visual signs require observation of actual movements. When the muscles and nerves become cooler, the participants' movements may become less strong, less energetic, and poorly co-ordinated.

## How can we encourage participants to stay warm?

We can maintain the warmth of participants by encouraging them to keep moving energetically throughout the session. By adding speed and strength to their movements they should be able to maintain a comfortable temperature. Session structure can also be adapted to promote warmth, and the exercises selected should be those that prevent unnecessary cooling of the body. It may well be necessary to include a longer warm-up, more active exercises and a shorter cool-down if working in a cooler pool.

However, the fitness level of the participants should also be considered prior to increasing the activity of the main workout and altering class structure too dramatically. An additional and equally effective alternative approach is to alternate the less active work of the smaller muscles with the more intense work of the larger muscles. This can assist with the generation of heat and assist the maintenance of a comfortable body temperature, without having to alter the session structure too much. Ideally, movements using a larger range of motion and of varying intensities should be performed throughout the whole session. This should accommodate different fitness levels safely and ensure that participants stay warm even throughout the slower and less energetic components of the session.

### NEED TO KNOW

**Summary of the effects of water temperature**

- Water has a cooling effect on the body.
- Constant movement is needed to assist the maintenance of a comfortable temperature when working in pools with a cooler temperature.
- We perspire less in water.
- If working in very hot pools, the intensity of the session should be lower and the duration shorter. We should re-hydrate regularly by drinking water.
- Leaner body types will cool down more quickly than fatter or more muscular body types.

# SUMMARY OF THE PROPERTIES OF WATER

Buoyancy, resistance and hydrostatic pressure provide many unique advantages to the exercising body. Their combined benefits are many, including:

- reduced stress placed on weight-bearing joints
- assisted movement of the body levers, which promotes the achievement of a larger range of motion
- added resistance to body movements, requiring greater muscular effort and calorie expenditure
- increased circulation of blood through the heart and body tissues, which decreases the stress on the heart muscle and promotes maximal use of the aerobic energy system to fuel movement
- decreased risk of blood pooling and improved return of venous blood to the heart.

It is clear that exercising in water provides us with many advantages. It is therefore an ideal medium for training a range of different populations, from the injured and unfit to trained athletes and sportspeople. However, the aforementioned properties need to be manipulated effectively to optimise the benefits that participants receive.

Knowledge of these watery effects is only one step towards designing an effective programme. A sound working knowledge of how the body works, and methods of training the body effectively are also of paramount importance. Chapter 2 introduces these concepts, which are explored further throughout the rest of the book. However, equally important is experience in water. Familiarise yourself with the effects of water by actually performing and rehearsing the water-based programmes. Such practice is essential for any prospective water-based exercise teacher: without sufficient experience in water they will not be sensitive to the effects of water on participants' movements. This may potentially render the programmes they design ineffective and possibly unsafe.

# SHORT ANSWER REVISION QUESTIONS

1. State **TWO** ways buoyancy will affect the body.

2. Give **TWO** examples of how body composition will influence buoyancy and levels of flotation.

3. Give **ONE** example of how body type may affect body composition and levels of buoyancy.

4. State **TWO** ways distribution of body fat will affect flotation.

5. Describe:
   (a) frontal resistance
   (b) eddy resistance
   (c) viscous resistance.

6. Describe the difference between concentric and eccentric muscle work.

7. Describe how frontal resistance will affect muscle contraction in a water-based session.

8. Describe how propulsive movements can be used to regain balance in a water-based session.

9. Describe how sculling techniques can be used to assist balance.

10. State **TWO** effects of hydrostatic pressure on the body systems.

11. State **TWO** ways water and air temperature will influence movement and exercise selection.

# THE BENEFITS OF
# WATER-BASED EXERCISE

2

## OBJECTIVES

By the end of this chapter the reader will be able to:

- Name the five components of physical fitness
- Name the body systems affected and improved by training each of the specific components of physical fitness
- Explain some of the benefits for improving each component of physical fitness
- Name the three major systems used to produce energy for activity and exercise
- Recognise the fuels used by each energy system
- Recognise activities that utilise each energy system
- Recognise the American College of Sports Medicine (ACSM 2006) training guidelines for improving each component of physical fitness
- Identify appropriate activities that may be included within an exercise in water session to improve each component of physical fitness
- Name and describe the components of total fitness
- Recognise the contribution of exercise in water (aqua) as a training mode for improving total fitness/health.

## What are the general benefits of water-based activities?

Exercise in water can improve physical fitness and promote a healthier lifestyle for a variety of different populations. The effects of the different properties of water provide many benefits to the submerged body. The reduced effects of gravity and increased effects of buoyancy provide support to the bodyweight and decrease the stress placed on the weight-bearing joints. This makes water-based activities a potentially safer and more comfortable form of training for specialist groups, such as the overweight, preg-

nant, senior, physically less able and injured participant. However, the extra resistance water provides to all movements can increase their intensity. This makes it an effective medium for training more general populations and sportspeople. Everyone can benefit from participating in a water-based exercise programme.

Well-designed water-based exercise programmes can improve all the components of fitness that contribute to the physical fitness of an individual. The components that are most essential for maintaining our fitness for life, and fitness to participate in sporting activities, are cardiovascular fitness, muscular strength, muscular endurance and flexibility. However, sportspeople will need additional training of more specific skill-related components that are referred to as motor fitness. These skill-related components include agility, balance, reaction time, speed, power and co-ordination.

Being physically fit will contribute to our overall health or total fitness. However, to be totally fit we need also to be socially, mentally, emotionally, nutritionally, spiritually and medically fit.

This chapter explores and discusses each of the components of physical and total fitness. It also identifies how water-based activities can contribute towards improving our physical fitness and lead us towards improved health, well-being and total fitness.

## What is cardiovascular fitness?

Cardiovascular fitness is the ability of the heart, lungs and circulatory system to transport and utilise oxygen efficiently, and remove waste products of aerobic and anaerobic energy production (carbon dioxide and lactic acid) with equal efficiency. It is sometimes referred to as cardio-respiratory fitness, stamina, or aerobic fitness.

Generally the more cardiovascular fitness an individual has (efficiency of the above processes), the higher will be their aerobic capacity or $VO_2$ max. This means they can work at a higher intensity (work level) and continue to provide oxygen (work aerobically) to meet the demands before the onset of blood lactate accumulation (OBLA) – anaerobic. This is discussed further in later paragraphs.

## Why do we need cardiovascular fitness?

A strong heart (cardiac muscle) and efficient respiratory and circulatory systems are essential for maintaining our quality of life and enabling our continued participation in sporting and recreational activities. A weak heart and inefficient respiratory and circulatory systems are more susceptible to diseases that cause premature death. Coronary heart disease is one of the highest causes of death in the Western world. Increased physical activity and improved cardiovascular fitness can assist with the prevention of such diseases. However, most recent White Papers issued by the Department of Health show evidence that physical activity levels are declining and coronary related diseases (high blood pressure, diabetes, high cholesterol) are increasing (DoH 2004, 2005).

The long-term benefits of specific training to improve this component will improve the efficiency of the heart, lungs and blood vessels. The heart will become stronger, which allows it to pump a greater volume of blood in each contraction (stroke volume). The capillary network in our muscles will also expand, which allows the transportation of more oxygen to the body cells and the swifter removal of waste products (lactic acid and carbon dioxide). The size and number of mitochondria, the cells in which aerobic energy is produced, will also increase, which in turn will enable us to deliver and utilise the oxygen that our muscles receive more effectively. Indeed, since oxygen is essential for our long-term production of energy, our performance of such activities will be enhanced. This will enable us to continue performing such activities for a more extended period of time.

Additionally, the activities that make demands on this system increase the metabolic rate (the rate at which we use energy or burn calories). Therefore, the frequent performance of the appropriate activities will assist with the reduction of body fat and the lowering of cholesterol levels, both of which will assist with effective weight management. The increased strength and efficiency of the cardiovascular system,

## SUMMARY OF THE LONG-TERM BENEFITS OF CARDIOVASCULAR TRAINING

- Stronger heart – cardiac muscle
- Increased stroke volume (amount of blood pumped in each contraction of the heart)
- Increased capillarisation (more blood vessels delivering blood and oxygen to the muscles and removing waste products from the muscles, which enables them to work for longer)
- Increased size and number of mitochondria (cells in which energy is produced aerobically – with oxygen)
- Increased metabolic rate (rate at which we burn calories)
- Decreased body fat
- Improved body composition
- Improved ratio of cholesterol (increased ratio of healthy cholesterol – high density lipoprotein (HDL) which helps to remove plaque from artery walls, and reduced ratio of low density lipoprotein (LDL) which sticks against artery walls)
- Normalised blood pressure
- Decreased risk of coronary heart disease.

coupled with the reduction in body fat and cholesterol levels, may also contribute to the normalising of elevated blood pressure and maintaining a healthy body composition/weight. All of this has a potentially positive effect on our health.

## How can we improve our cardiovascular fitness?

To improve the fitness of the heart, respiratory and circulatory systems, we need to perform rhythmical activities that use the larger muscles of the body. These should be performed on a regular basis, ideally between three and five times per week. The activities should be performed at a moderate intensity to create a feeling of mild breathlessness without making us feel any unnecessary discomfort. We should be able to sustain these activities comfortably for a prolonged duration. Traditional activities that promote this type of fitness are walking, running, cycling, aerobic dancing, rowing, swimming etc. Adherence to this type of exercise programme will induce the necessary long-term health-related improvements to the cardiovascular system. The recommended training requirements for improvements of cardiovascular fitness are outlined in table 2.1 on page 31.

As a starting point, inactive individuals who wish to build their physical activity levels to maintain general health are advised to follow the Department of Health (2004 and 2005) guidelines (*see* table 2.2 on page 32) and work towards the ACSM (2006) targets (*see* table 2.1). The DoH (2005) targets are currently under review, as to whether they are sufficient to reduce health risks.

| Table 2.1 | The recommended training requirements for improving cardiovascular fitness | |
|---|---|
| Frequency How often? | 3–5 times a week (decrease frequency when working at higher intensity). Ideally vary the activities to prevent overuse of specific body areas. |
| Intensity How hard? | Between 55–65% and 90% maximal heart rate with different target heart rate zones being used to indicate the working level for different training goals and individual fitness. |
| | Equivalent to Rate of Perceived Exertion (RPE) 12–16 (somewhat hard to hard). NB: Exercise intensity is explored further in chapter 5. |
| | 50–60% of Maximum Heart Rate (MHR) for improving health of untrained individuals. |
| | 60–70% of MHR for assisting weight management. NB: Lower intensity can be sustained for longer and increased duration is often a recommendation for weight management programmes. |
| | 70–80% of MHR for developing a base level of cardiovascular fitness from which future training goals can progress. |
| | 80–90% of MHR for improving cardiovascular fitness of highly trained individuals to peak performance levels. Onset of blood lactate (OBLA) zone. |
| | 90–100% for anaerobic performance zone. |
| Time How long? | Between 20 and 60 minutes of continuous or intermittent activity (10 minute bouts accumulated throughout the day). With a minimum of 20 minutes to develop aerobic capacity. |
| Type | Any exercise that uses large muscle groups of the body and which can be performed continuously for the sustained duration. For example: running, swimming, cycling, rowing. |

Adapted from: American College of Sports Medicine (ACSM) 2006

| Table 2.2 | Physical activity targets – five times per week | | |
|---|---|---|---|
| Frequency | Build physical activity into daily routine **five days per week** (minimum) | | |
| Intensity | Work to a moderate level where you **feel mildly breathless, warm but comfortable** (Level 3–4 on Borg's CR-10 intensity scale) | | |
| Time | Be active for **30 minutes** on each of the five days. This can be broken down and accumulated, for example:<br>**3 x 10** minute slots of activity each day<br>**2 x 15** minute slots of activity each day | | |
| Type | Any activity that fits well into your daily lifestyle!<br><br>For example:<br>• Walking instead of driving or using other transport<br>• Vigorous housework<br>• Cleaning the car, instead of using the car wash<br>• Walking up and down stairs more frequently<br>• Dancing to a piece of music at home<br>• Structured exercise and sporting activities (badminton etc).<br><br>These recommendations can be tailored specifically to the lifestyle, preference and needs of the individual and are particularly relevant for people who find it easier and more acceptable to increase physical activity by incorporating it into their everyday life. | | |

Source: Department of Health (2004, 2005)

## How do we provide energy for activity to improve cardiovascular fitness?

In order for our bodies to function, perform daily tasks and participate in exercise or activity to improve physical fitness, the body has to create energy. This energy comes in the form of a chemical called Adenosine Tri Phosphate (ATP), which is only stored in limited amounts and needs continually to be replenished to create energy to sustain activity and life. ATP derives from the breakdown (via digestion) of the nutrients (carbohydrates, fats and protein) we obtain from our diet.

During periods of inactivity, energy demands are lower and the heart, lungs and circulatory system (if healthy) can usually supply the necessary oxygen to replenish ATP and maintain functioning. During exercise and activity the physiological demands increase and so too are the demands for ATP production to sustain the increased workload. Other systems are needed to cater for times when demands for oxygen cannot be met immediately by the cardiovascular system.

ATP is replenished by the following energy systems in the body:
- The creatine phosphate system – anaerobic (without oxygen).
- The glycogen or lactic acid system – anaerobic (without oxygen).
- The oxygen system – aerobic (with oxygen).

The main factors that determine which energy system is used to re-synthesise ATP are:
- Intensity of the activity – how hard is it?
- Duration of the activity – how long is it performed for?
- Fitness level of the person performing the activity.
- Skill level of the person performing the activity, that is, how familiar they are with performing that activity (specificity).

## Creatine phosphate system

Creatine phosphate provides an immediately available source for replenishing ATP stores. It is stored in limited amounts in the muscles and is used for immediate bursts of activity and explosive activities that can only be sustained for a short duration (no more than 6–10 seconds). It would be used predominately during 100m sprints, power lifting, long jump and high jump events.

Within a water-based session, activities that may challenge this system include explosive movements such as tuck jumps that lift the body out of the water at a rapid pace. Rest intervals between these higher intensity exercises will need to be longer to enable replenishment of ATP-CP stores and to reduce the accumulation of lactic acid.

## Glycogen/lactic acid system

Glycogen is the next readily available energy source that is stored in the liver and muscles and can be broken down to reform ATP. The glycogen system is used predominantly during high intensity activities that usually last for no longer than between 60 and 180 seconds. Athletic track events that use this energy system would be the 400 and 800 metres.

The limiting factor of this system is the accumulation of lactic acid that builds up during the breakdown of glycogen without the presence of oxygen. When lactic acid accumulates, it contributes to fatigue and is experienced as a burning sensation in the muscles. Exercise intensity will need to decrease or be stopped to assist removal of lactic acid via the circulatory system.

According to McArdle et al (1991:125): 'Lactic acid begins to accumulate and rise in an exponential fashion at about 55 per cent of the healthy, untrained subject's maximal capacity ($VO_2$ max) for aerobic metabolism'. As exercise intensity increases, so too does the level of lactic acid. For trained individuals, the accumulation of lactic acid generally occurs at a higher level of their maximal capacity ($VO_2$ max). Trained endurance athletes frequently perform at intensities equivalent to between 80 and 90 per cent of their maximal capacity ($VO_2$ max). This indicates that the level at which the onset of blood lactate (OBLA) occurs can be improved through training (see discussion within aerobic energy system, for physiological adaptations to aerobic training that may contribute to OBLA occurring at higher exercise intensities).

The point at which lactic acid accumulates – the blood lactate threshold – is commonly referred to as the anaerobic threshold.

## Oxygen system

The aerobic or oxygen system takes a little longer to engage than the other systems during exercise and activity. This is because other physiological processes need to occur to circulate oxygen to meet the demands; the heart rate and breathing rate need to increase to take in and circulate oxygen, and the blood vessels need to dilate to allow the uptake of oxygen. In addition, there will need to be sufficient cells in the muscle (mitochondria) to enable ATP replenishment and aerobic energy production. However, the major advantage of this system is that greater amounts of ATP can be produced and these increased levels can be maintained for longer durations when working at a steady state. In addition, the waste products – carbon dioxide, heat and water – are comparatively easy for the body to remove through exhalation and sweating.

The aerobic or oxygen system uses a combination of nutrients (carbohydrates, fats and protein), which are broken down in the presence of oxygen (aerobic) to replenish ATP stored and to sustain activity. Activities that use the aerobic system are those that can be maintained for a longer duration but at a lower to moderate intensity. Athletic events such as the marathon and other long distance endurance running, swimming and cycling events would use this system predominantly.

The long-term effects of regular aerobic cardiovascular training include increased size and number of mitochondria and increased capillaries within the muscles. These adaptations enable more oxygen to be delivered and used by the muscles for energy production. They also enable the more effective removal of waste products that accumulate (lactic acid). These muscular adaptations are cited as being potentially responsible for the later onset of blood lactate accumulation (OBLA) among trained individuals, when working at higher levels of intensity. This means trained individuals can work at higher levels before the onset of blood lactate occurs.

A further benefit is that the body becomes more efficient in utilising its fat stores. Aerobic cardiovascular training is often a key prescriptive feature within weight management and fat loss training programmes.

## How will the energy systems engage during a water-based session?

During a water-based session the energy systems will interweave. At different times, different energy systems may be more dominant depending on the intensity and duration of the activity, and the fitness level of the individual performing the activity.

At the start of the session, all systems will be activated, with the anaerobic systems being most active, until the circulatory system has time to respond to the warming up activities. If the intensity of the preparatory phase is appropriate, the aerobic system will become the predominant system. If the intensity of the warm-up is too high, exercise intensity will need to reduce to maximise the aerobic system.

During the main workout, the intensity of specific exercises and the fitness level of the individual will determine the energy system used. High intensity exercises will potentially challenge the anaerobic system, whereas lower intensity stations and recovery periods will allow the aerobic system to be utilised predominately. A key consideration with exercise in water, however, is the hydrostatic pressure. This provides assistance to the circulatory system and may therefore reduce the extent to which the body will work using anaerobic systems when exercising in water. Hydrostatic pressure is discussed in Chapter 1.

| Table 2.3 | Energy system summary | | |
|---|---|---|---|
| Energy System | Creatine Phosphate | Lactic acid/Glycogen | Oxygen |
| Fuel used | Creatine phosphate | Glycogen | Glycogen, fat protein |
| ATP production | Very limited | Limited | Unlimited |
| Engagement | Very rapid – immediate | Rapid | Slow (cardiovascular system needs to engage to circulate blood/oxygen) |
| Muscle fibre | Fast twitch | Fast oxidative glycolytic (FOG) | Slow twitch |
| Fuel stored | Muscles | Muscles and liver | Glycogen stored in muscle. Fat stored as adipose tissue |
| Amounts of fuel available | Limited. Only a few seconds | Moderate supply. From few seconds to up to 2–3 minutes | Glycogen moderate. Fat more plentiful. System can sustain activity for as long as fuel available |
| Intensity, duration and type of activity | High intensity Short duration 100m sprint Throwing and jumping events Strength training | Moderate to high intensity 400m sprint Anaerobic endurance (8–25 repetitions approximately) | Low to moderate intensity. Longer duration. Marathon running. Long distance swimming and cycling. Circuit weight training |
| Waste products | Creatine | Lactic acid accumulation inhibits muscle contraction. | Carbon dioxide – exhaled. Heat generated, body produces water/sweat to regulate temperature |
| Limitations | Short supply of creatine phosphate | Lactic acid build-up | Takes longer to engage |

Adapted from: Lawrence & Hope (2007)

| Table 2.4 | Energy systems used in different sporting activities | |
|---|---|---|
| Sporting events | Aerobic – with oxygen (%) | Anaerobic – without oxygen (%) |
| Marathon run | 100 | 0 |
| 400m swim<br>Rowing 2000m | 60–70 | 30–40 |
| Water polo, hockey, netball, football, rugby game<br><br>NB: Position of player and activity levels will affect energy systems used | 50 | 50 |
| 800m run | 40 | 60 |
| 100m swim | 20 | 80 |
| 100m sprint | 0 | 100 |

Adapted with reference from: Davis, Roscoe, Roscoe, Bull (2005) & Davis, Kimmet, Auty (1986)

## What types of activities are appropriate for a water-based session?

The traditional land-based activities that improve cardiovascular fitness, such as running and cycling, require greater use of the lower body and minimal work of the upper body. Alternatively, the traditional water-based activities to improve this component of fitness, such as swimming and rowing, require the upper body to have a much greater involvement. Swimming is advocated by many as the most holistic mode of training, appropriate for everybody. This is perhaps because it utilises a larger proportion of the muscles and is supportive to the body. Other water-based exercise techniques can provide an equally holistic approach. This is, of course, provided the activities are well selected and structured.

The most effective types of water-based exercises to bring about the desired training benefits, and improve this component of fitness, are those that require us to move our centre of gravity/ buoyancy through the water. Movements that require us to jump out of the water, and movements which require us to travel through the water, are very effective (*see* Fig. 2.1).

Explosive leaping movements require plenty of muscular effort to move our centre of buoyancy and lift our bodyweight out of the water. As we return into the water, the surface tension of the water creates further resistance to our

## Fig. 2.1 — Movement of the centre of buoyancy/gravity during jumping and travelling movements

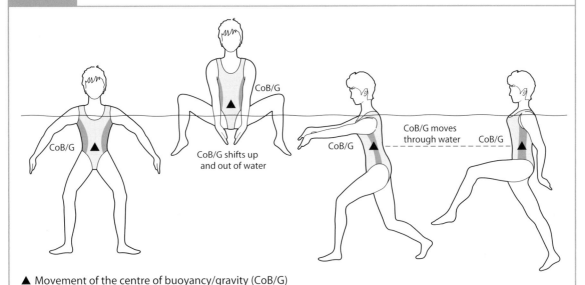

▲ Movement of the centre of buoyancy/gravity (CoB/G)

Note: Jumping out of the water lifts the weight of the body and centre of buoyancy through a larger range of motion. Travelling through the water will also increase the range of motion through which the centre of buoyancy moves. The latter will additionally require strong propulsive movements to move the body against the resistance of the water.

body and its movement back down through the water surface to the pool floor. This slows down our movement and makes it harder for us to regain the balance and momentum to repeat the movement. These activities are much safer when performed in water due to the support provided by buoyancy. They are far more controversial when performed on land, due to the increased force borne by the joints. However, they are still very intense when performed in water and can generally only be comfortably sustained for a shorter duration of time. They should therefore be combined with other more moderately paced activities.

Travelling movements require us to use strong propulsive actions to shift our body mass through the water. This maximises the use of the different resistances provided by the water, and therefore requires us to exert more muscular effort to create such movements and maintain balance. Travelling movements are therefore potentially the most effective way of increasing and sustaining the intensity of the workout, and thus of improving cardiovascular fitness.

Strong movements of the upper body under the water will also be very effective. The added resistance that water provides to movement will create equally demanding work for the muscles of the back, chest, and arms when they are moving under the water. Therefore large movements of the upper body that require these muscles to pull, drag and push against the resistance of the water will also be very effective.

## Will moving the arms out of the water be effective?

Lifting and using the arms out of the water is a less effective method of training to improve cardiovascular fitness. These movements will increase the heart rate because the heart will have to work harder to pump the blood upwards against the pull of gravity. However, they will not demand such an effective uptake of oxygen. This is because the muscles primarily responsible for performing such movements (deltoids, biceps, trapezius, etc.) are comparatively smaller than the larger leg muscles. When they work out of the water against gravity they are presented with little resistance to their movement, much less than when they are working underneath the water surface and against the resistance of the water. In addition, continuous arm work above the head and out of the water may have an adverse effect on blood pressure, which is neither desired nor recommended.

## How can different fitness levels be catered for?

The intensity of activities selected should correspond to the fitness level of participants. The activities selected for a less fit person need to be of a lower intensity. This is because their heart will have to work somewhat harder to deliver the same volume of blood and their muscles will be less efficient at making effective use of the oxygen they receive. Therefore, very intense movements should be adapted to make them less intense. This can be achieved by using shorter levers, slower movements, comparatively less travelling, and by exerting less force when performing each movement.

In addition, while explosive movements are safer when performed in water, they are not highly recommended for those with a very low level of fitness or those with specialist requirements. This is because such activities require a greater body awareness and strong muscular fixation to be performed effectively, and for safe alignment to be maintained. Ultimately, there are much safer alternative types of activities that are equally effective, potentially safer, and far easier to perform correctly and with safe alignment.

Alternatively, fitter participants will need to be challenged. Their heart will be stronger and able to supply oxygen with less effort, and their muscles will make more effective use of the oxygen delivered. Therefore, they should be encouraged to put greater effort into all of their movements and can be encouraged to jump and travel more frequently during the programme. They should also be encouraged to use longer levers and faster movements more regularly. It is easier for them to cheat in water, so they should be encouraged to apply greater force to their movements and work the water for maximum effect.

Explosive movements in water will be much safer when performed by fitter participants. Firstly, their body awareness and skill levels should be greater, and secondly their muscles should be stronger. Both these factors will promote the maintenance of correct alignment and form, enhancing the safety of any exercise.

## What is flexibility?

Flexibility is the ability of our joints and muscles to move through their full potential range of movement. It is sometimes referred to as suppleness and mobility.

# Why do we need flexibility?

The ability of the joints and muscles to move through their full potential range of motion is essential for easing the performance of everyday tasks. We need flexibility in our shoulder joint to reach above our head and change a light bulb, or to reach for an object on a high shelf. We need flexibility in our hip joint to climb stairs, and take long strides when walking. If we are flexible we can move more efficiently.

In addition, flexible joints and muscles will contribute to the maintenance of correct posture and joint alignment. Improved posture can potentially enhance our physical appearance. Indeed, standing tall and upright can have a slimming effect on most body frames. Therefore, being sufficiently flexible will allow us to move with greater ease, and with greater poise.

Conversely, a lack of flexibility will cause our bodies to become stiff and immobile. We will be less able to reach up to a high shelf, and less able to bend down and tie our shoe laces. This can restrict the everyday movements we are able to perform, and make us less self-sufficient. In addition, moving around with an incorrect posture and joint alignment will potentially create muscle imbalance, and possibly increase our risk of injury. Poor posture will also create a less aesthetically pleasing appearance. Therefore, being flexible is of paramount impor-

tance for improving the quality and economy of our movements in everyday life.

Being sufficiently flexible will also contribute to the enhancement of our performance during sporting and recreational activities. If we are not sufficiently flexible, we are more susceptible to injury, especially when performing activities that require us to move quickly into extended positions, such as bending down, reaching up and away, and twisting around. However, some sporting activities require much more flexibility than we need to perform our daily tasks. In particular, some of the martial arts and dance activities require excessive flexibility. These activities can lead to us having too much flexibility. If we are too flexible, and the muscles and ligaments around the joint are not strong enough to keep the joint stable, we are also promoting greater risk of injury.

Ultimately, we need the right amount of flexibility to perform our everyday tasks, and maintain correct alignment. However, if we participate in sporting activities we may require a little extra. A competitive sportsperson and professional dancer will need greater flexibility to assist with the achievement of their goals. However, if we participate in sporting activities for recreational purposes, it is arguable whether we should push ourselves so far. The key issue is to decide our reasons for participating, and our individual aims. Ideally, we

---

## SUMMARY OF THE LONG-TERM BENEFITS OF FLEXIBILITY TRAINING

- Improved range of motion in the joints and muscles
- Improved posture and joint alignment
- Potential for enhanced exercise technique, and the performance of sporting and everyday activities
- Reduced tension in the muscles
- Reduced risk of injury when moving into extended positions.

should ensure that we are flexible enough to meet the demands placed on our body, without placing our bodies at risk from injury.

## How can we improve flexibility?

Flexibility can be maintained by the frequent (daily) performance of activities that require our muscles and joints to move through their full range of motion. Since most sedentary lifestyles do not naturally provide this opportunity, stretching activities are incorporated into most fitness programmes.

**Stretching** activities are those which require the two ends of the muscle, the origin and insertion, to move further apart. This causes the muscle to lengthen, and will potentially increase the range of motion at the joint. However, the muscle must also be allowed to relax to achieve an effective stretch.

**Static stretch** positions are generally advocated as safer for most individuals in land-based exercise sessions. Static stretches require comfortable supportive positions to be adopted and held still for an appropriate duration. The aim is to enable the tension initially felt in the muscle (the stretch reflex) to dissipate (de-sensitisation) and allow the muscle to relax and move more safely to an extended range of movement. However, if we move too quickly or too far into the stretch (overstretching), then relaxation of the stretch reflex may not occur. It is therefore essential that we listen carefully to our body and move only to the point of a mild, initial discomfort. A disadvantage of performing these stretches in water is that the body will cool down quickly, and muscles should be warm to stretch.

**Active stretching** is where the opposite muscle contracts to bring about a stretch of the other muscle pair. For example: contracting the hip flexor to raise the knee upwards would be an active stretch of the gluteals. The disadvantage of active stretching is that the positions are sometimes less relaxing. In the example described, the hip flexor would work statically (isometric) to hold the position; over a period of time this would increase tension in the hip flexor muscle, reduce oxygen delivered to the muscle, and potentially contribute to lactic acid building up in the muscle (hip flexor). The stretch would need to be released to remove these effects.

**Passive stretching** is where both the prime mover/agonist and antagonist relax. This is achieved by supporting the stretch position. Passive stretching potentially enables more relaxation. For example: to stretch the gluteals, raise the knee in front of the body and hold with the hands. This enables the hip flexor to relax, so both muscles can relax. The stretch position can usually be maintained for longer. Fig. 2.2 on page 4 indicates how water assists with relaxation of the opposite muscle.

**Ballistic stretching movements** are discouraged in most health-related exercise sessions. Ballistic stretches are those that require the body to move too quickly into an extended range of motion. They tend to maintain activity of the stretch reflex and prevent de-sensitisation occurring. In addition, the momentum produced may potentially cause the range of motion to be exceeded and create a risk of muscle tearing and damage to the ligaments and other tissues that surround the joint. In the long term such activities may reduce stability of the joints, creating hyper-mobility. They may cause irreparable damage to the muscles and joints, which may restrict range of motion and decrease flexibility.

Another method of stretching, that is sometimes recommended (particularly for water-based programmes) is **dynamic or range of motion stretching**. Dynamic stretching occurs when the joints and muscles move through the full range of motion but there is no specific static holding phase. The movement into and out of the extended range is continued for a specific number of repetitions. These stretches can be performed fairly safely in water because the resistance of the water prevents the speed of movement becoming ballistic in nature.

| Table 2.5 | The recommended training requirements for improving flexibility |
|---|---|
| Frequency How often? | 2–3 times per week minimum. 5–7 times per week is ideal. NB: The muscles must be warm prior to stretching to prevent muscle tearing and promote range of motion. |
| Intensity How hard? | Positions that promote the feeling of mild tension/tightness (not pain) in the belly of the muscle at the end of the range of movement. 2–4 repetitions of each stretch can be performed. |
| Time How long? | Static stretching – 15–30 seconds hold. PNF (proprioceptive neuromuscular facilitation) stretching – 6 second contract followed by 10–30 second assisted stretch. |
| Type | Static or PNF techniques for all major muscle groups. Slow and controlled performance progressing to greater ranges of movement. It is also essential to give consideration to the specific flexibility needs of the individuals (current flexibility levels and flexibility needs for their specific sporting activity). Adapted from: ACSM (2000:158) and ACSM (2006:162) |
| Exercise in water considerations | PNF stretching is not appropriate for water-based sessions and the water temperature would need to be very warm for the inclusion of a lot of static stretching. It is recommended and discussed in subsequent paragraphs that dynamic range of motion stretches are used for water-based programmes. |

## NEED TO KNOW

**The stretch reflex** forms part of the Peripheral Nervous System (PNS). It can be described as a safety mechanism to prevent over-stretching. This propriceptor is stimulated when the muscle changes length and registers the speed of movement and amount of lengthening or stretch that is occurring and relays this to the Central Nervous System. The CNS informs the muscle being lengthened to contract (the feeling of tension that is felt in the muscle), to prevent injury to the muscle and surrounding tissues.

**Fig. 2.2** **Buoyancy assisting the performance of a stretch for the muscles at the back of the thigh**

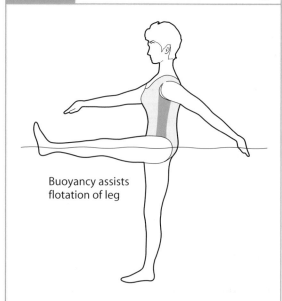

Buoyancy assists flotation of leg

## How can exercising in water improve our range of motion and flexibility?

The buoyancy of the water can be used to support the body and promote more passive stretching. If we allow our limbs to float to the surface of the water, the muscles that are normally required to contract and hold such positions are able to relax. This reduces the tension and activity (active stretching) in these muscles and allows us to achieve a fuller range of motion of most joint areas quite naturally, making the stretch positions more passive in nature. One example of this is to allow the leg to rise and float in front of the body to stretch the muscles at the back of the thigh (the hamstring – *see* Fig. 2.2).

Additionally, the frontal resistance exerted by the water will restrict the speed of our movements and will prevent the natural range of motion being exceeded. There will be less risk of these movements becoming ballistic.

Note: On land, the muscles at the front of the thigh and hip (quadriceps and hip flexors) would have to contract very strongly to hold this position. The height of the movement achieved would be limited by the strength of these muscles, and the opposing muscle groups at the back of the thigh and buttocks (hamstrings and gluteals) would lengthen minimally, providing an, albeit limited, active stretch of these muscles. In water, the leg will float and can generally rise much higher. The muscles at the front of the thigh should be able to relax and be supported by the water (this will depend on the body composition of the performer). Ultimately, a greater range of motion should be achieved because the water will allow the muscles to relax, and thus creates what is referred to as a passive stretch – the opposing muscle to the one targeted to be stretched is able to relax.

Therefore, the performance of more flowing and relaxed movements that allow the muscles to reach the end of their range of motion slowly (dynamic/moving stretches), are potentially safer in water since less risk of injury is attached. Moving each joint area as far as you can, under the water, and in all possible directions will improve their range of motion. These movements can replace many of the necessary static stretches required to move safely to an extended range of motion on land. In addition, they will assist with the maintenance of a comfortable body temperature if exercising in cooler pool temperatures.

A higher proportion of static stretches is only recommended when working in warmer pool temperatures. However, if static stretches are preferred, then the inclusion of a larger proportion of movements to keep warm between stretches will be necessary to maintain a comfortable body temperature. This will also ensure that the muscles are sufficiently warm to move to an extended range of motion. Performing static stretches in cooler pool temperatures, without sufficient activities to maintain warmth, are potentially unsafe since the muscles will be less elastic and more at risk from injury when moving to an extended range of motion. In addition, the use of the poolside and/or the use of sculling movements of the arm will be necessary to assist with the maintenance of a balanced and stable position during the performance of some static stretches.

Ultimately, a combination of the two types of stretches is recommended. Dynamic/moving stretches for the normally flexible muscles are sufficient to prepare muscles prior to work, and maintain range of motion after work. However, the muscles which are normally less flexible due to our sedentary lifestyles, for example the hamstrings, hip flexors and adductors, are perhaps more likely to benefit from static stretches. In addition, if working with less flex-ible groups they are arguably potentially much safer, even when working in the pool.

## How can we cater for different levels of flexibility?

Less flexible participants will generally need to work through a smaller range of motion. It is much easier to control their range of motion by using static stretches. However, body temperature needs to be monitored! Static stretches will assist with preventing them exceeding a safe range of motion. They should only move into a stretch position to a point where they feel a mild tension. This may require some stretch positions to be adapted so they are able to stay within a comfortable range. If dynamic/range of motion/moving stretches are used with the less skilled or flexible, they should be advised only to move to a point where they feel comfortable. Their movements throughout the main workout will also need to be slightly smaller and perhaps slower. It may be necessary for them to perform movements with shorter levers and a smaller range of motion to prevent them from overstretching.

More flexible participants should be able to move quite safely through a larger range of motion. They should be encouraged to use longer levers and fully extend (straighten) their joints, without locking them (hyper-extending), to move to their full potential. Potentially, the majority of their stretches can be dynamic/range of motion, provided the participants have sufficient body awareness and muscular control of their movements.

## What is muscular strength and endurance?

Muscular strength is the ability of our muscles to exert a near maximal force to lift a resistance

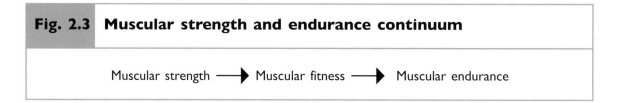

**Fig. 2.3** **Muscular strength and endurance continuum**

Muscular strength ⟶ Muscular fitness ⟶ Muscular endurance

(training with high resistance for low repetitions). Muscular endurance requires a less maximal force to be exerted, but maintained for a longer duration (training with lower resistance for higher repetitions). They each represent polar ends of a continuum. Muscular fitness (a combination of strength and endurance) represents an optimal level of fitness for functional and health-related purposes.

## Why do we need muscular strength and muscular endurance?

Our muscles need to be strong enough and have sufficient endurance to carry out daily tasks that require us to lift, carry, pull, or push a resistance. This may include shopping, gardening, moving furniture, climbing stairs and lifting ourselves out of a chair or bath. If we participate in sporting activities, either recreationally or competitively, then we may require greater strength and endurance than we normally need to perform our daily tasks efficiently. In daily life we never need to lift the heavy weights a power lifter would need to move. Neither do we need the endurance to perform thousands of press-ups or sit-ups. Our primary aim should therefore be that our muscles are strong enough to perform our daily tasks, perhaps with a little in reserve.

Strong muscles will help us to maintain the correct alignment of our skeleton, but weak muscles may cause an uneven pull to be placed on our skeleton. Our muscles work in pairs –

as one contracts and works (prime mover or agonist), the opposite muscle (antagonist) relaxes. Therefore, if one of the pair is contracted or worked too frequently and becomes too strong and the other is not worked sufficiently or is allowed to become weaker, then our joints will be pulled out of the correct alignment. This may potentially cause injury, or create postural defects such as rounded shoulders or excessive curvatures of the spine (*see* Fig. 2.4).

### NEED TO KNOW

Muscles work in pairs and pull on bones (levers) to bring about movement
- Prime mover/agonist – main muscle contracting to bring about a movement.
- Antagonist – opposite muscle to prime mover that relaxes as prime mover contracts.
- Fixator – muscle contracting to hold other joints in alignment during the movement (fix the origin of the prime mover).
- Synergist – assistant to prime mover or contracts to hold other joints in alignment during movement (fix the insertion of the prime mover). Tyldesley & Grieve (1989).

An imbalance of strength between the abdominal and opposing muscles of the back (the erector spinae) can cause an exaggerated curve or hollowing of the lumbar vertebrae (lordosis). An imbalance of strength between the muscles of the chest (the pectorals) and the muscles between the shoulder blades (the rhomboids and trapezius) can cause rounded shoulders and a humping of the thoracic spine (kyphosis). An imbalance in strength between the muscles on each side of the back can cause a sideways curvature of the thoracic spine (scoliosis).

All our muscles should therefore be kept sufficiently strong to maintain a correct posture. However, our lifestyle may demand that we specifically target certain muscles more than others. This is to compensate for the imbalances caused by our work and daily activities. For the majority of people with a sedentary lifestyle, it is well worth strengthening the abdominal muscles and the muscles in between the shoulder blades (trapezius and rhomboids).

### NEED TO KNOW

- Muscles can contract and get shorter to lift against a resistance – concentric.
- Muscles can contract and get longer to yield with a resistance – eccentric.
- Muscles can contract and stay the same length to hold a position – isometric/static.

Training for muscular strength and endurance will also improve the tone of our muscles. Toned

---

**Fig. 2.4** **Curvatures of the spine**

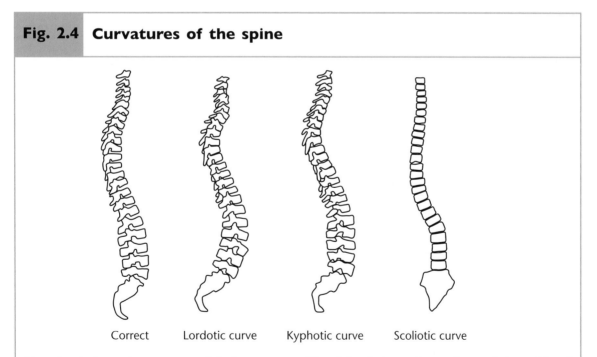

Correct  Lordotic curve  Kyphotic curve  Scoliotic curve

Note: Lordosis can be exaggerated during pregnancy. The abdominal muscles weaken and the weight of the baby can create a forward tilt of the pelvis. This places a lot of stress on the lumbar vertebrae. Kyphosis can be caused by slumping over a desk all day, and also possibly by driving. Scoliosis can be exaggerated by continuously carrying a bag or shopping using the same side of the body.

muscles are firmer and more shapely. Therefore, they can provide us with an improved body shape and physical appearance. If our body is toned and taut we may have a more positive self-image. This, in turn, can enhance our psychological well-being and self-confidence.

Finally, muscular strength and endurance training can also improve the strength and health of our bones and joints. The muscles have to contract and pull against the bones to create movement and lift the resistance. In response, our tendons, which attach the muscles to the bone across the joint, and our ligaments, which attach bone to bone across the joint, will become stronger. Therefore, in the long term our joints will become stronger, more stable, and at less risk from injury. In addition, increased calcium can be deposited and stored by the bones. This can prevent them from becoming brittle and reduce the risk of osteoporosis. Muscular strength and endurance training can therefore provide many long-lasting benefits, which can extend the quality of our life for a number of years.

## How do we improve our strength and endurance?

Strength training is traditionally achieved by performing exercises that require us to lift heavy and near maximal resistances for a short period of time (high resistance and low repetitions). Endurance exercises require a lighter resistance to be lifted but for an extended period of time (lower resistance and higher repetitions).

The type of activities that promote strength and endurance gains are those which require a more isolated focus on the specific muscles. Weight training is a typical training mode, although callisthenic exercises that require us to lift our bodyweight (such as press-ups, sit-ups, etc.) can be equally effective. These activities need to be performed approximately two to three times a week on non-consecutive days for sufficient improvement to be made. The resistance lifted should promote a fatigued feeling in the muscle at the end of the desired repetition range to achieve overload. Obviously the gains achieved by an individual will be determined by the number of repetitions they are able to perform. The lower the number of reps an individual is able to perform, the more the gains will be to muscular strength. The more repetitions an individual is able to perform, the more the gains will be to muscular endurance. The recommended training requirements for improving our muscular strength and muscular endurance are outlined in table 2.6 on page 48.

### NEED TO KNOW

Summary of the long-term benefits of muscular strength and endurance training
- Increased bone density (more calcium laid down).
- Decreased risk of osteoporosis – brittle bones.
- Improved posture and alignment.
- Improved performance of sporting and recreational activities.
- Efficient performance of daily tasks.
- Improved body shape and tone.
- Improved self-image.
- Improved self-confidence.
- Stronger muscles, ligaments and tendons which are more supportive to movement.

### NEED TO KNOW

- Strength – heavy resistance for lower repetitions.
- Endurance – lower resistance for higher repetitions.

## How can exercising in water improve our muscular strength and endurance?

Water exerts a resistance to our movements, which is approximately 12 times the resistance of air. This potentially provides us with a greater opportunity to overload and challenge the muscles. The majority of fitness gains will tend to be primarily for muscular endurance. This is because the resistance of water is still comparatively lower than that potentially lifted during a weight-training programme. However, this is dependent on the fitness level of the participants. Less fit or previously sedentary people may find the resistance of water sufficient to overload and improve both their muscular strength and endurance. Fitter participants, on the other hand, may need to use flotation devices to add further resistance and provide sufficient challenge. Exercises that use equipment are illustrated in Chapter 11.

While exercise in water will still provide the necessary improvements to muscular strength and endurance, it may be less effective at improving the density of our bones. This is because weight-bearing activities are generally the most effective to bring about these adaptations, and water-based exercising is considered non-weight bearing due to the support that buoyancy provides to the body. However, there may still be some improvements, because the muscles are contracting against a resistance to pull on the bones. Ultimately, improvements in bone density may be lower when exercising in water, but further research is needed into this area before conclusions are made.

### NEED TO KNOW

- Weight-bearing activities are most effective for improving bone density and reducing the risk of osteoporosis.
- Water-based exercise is considered non-weight bearing. The buoyancy of the water supports the weight of the body.

## How can different abilities be catered for?

Muscular strength and endurance activities can be intensified progressively by increasing the surface area of the body parts being moved, moving at a slightly faster pace, and exerting greater force. Less fit participants should be encouraged to progress more steadily by using these methods singularly.

Fitter participants can be encouraged to use all three of these progressive methods, which should provide them with a sufficient challenge. The use of flotation equipment will further increase the intensity of activities. The use of such devices may well be sufficient to challenge strength for a fitter group, but the use of equipment may be inappropriate for less fit participants. Their progression to working out at this level of intensity should be gradual – over a number of weeks, or possibly months.

Methods for increasing surface area are discussed in Chapter 1. Equipment that can increase surface area and add to buoyancy is discussed in Chapter 11.

| Table 2.6 | The recommended training requirements for improving muscular strength and endurance |
| --- | --- |
| Frequency | 2–3 days a week for the same muscle groups on non-consecutive days. More frequent training and increased sets, resistance and/or repetitions are appropriate for trained individuals with specific fitness goals. |
| Intensity | Minimum guidelines:<br>1 set of 3–20 reps (3–5, 8–10, 12–15)<br><br>8–12 repetitions to point of volitional fatigue.<br><br>Increased repetitions for muscular endurance with lighter resistance (10–15 repetitions +).<br><br>Increased resistance for muscular strength with lower repetitions (maximal or sub-maximal resistance recommended – 1– 6/8 RM Repetition Maximum).<br><br>8–10 exercises covering all muscle groups exercising whole body (back, arms, legs, abdominals, chest, hips, shoulders).<br><br>Full range of motion – isotonic.<br><br>Moderate to slow speed to enable concentric and eccentric control. Caution advised when focusing on eccentric contraction due to increased muscle soreness. |
| Time | 1 hour maximum duration to promote adherence.<br><br>Adapted from ACSM (2000) and ACSM (2007) |
| Type | Correct exercise technique.<br>Correct breathing to minimise potential for increases in blood pressure.<br><br>**In water:**<br>Use of surface area to add resistance to body movements.<br>Use of buoyancy equipment to add resistance (see Chapter 11).<br>Varying the speed of movements.<br>Pushing and pulling with greater force against the resistance of the water. |

## What is motor fitness?

Motor fitness is primarily a skill-related component of fitness and refers to a number of interrelated factors. The skill-related components of fitness include agility, balance, speed, co-ordination, reaction time and power.

## Why do we need motor fitness?

Motor fitness requires the effective transmission and management of messages and responses between the central nervous system (the brain and spinal cord) and the peripheral nervous system (sensory and motor). The peripheral system collects information via the sensory system; the central nervous system receives and processes this information and sends an appropriate response via the motor system, which initiates the appropriate response.

Motor fitness is perhaps more applicable to the sportsperson. However, it can have an indirect effect on the improvement of our fitness in the other health-related fitness components. Development of specific skills can improve our performance of certain activities. Skilful movements are more efficient: if we move skilfully we can improve the effectiveness of the activities we perform. In addition, by learning to perform exercises with the correct technique, we will reduce the risk of injury that can be caused by moving with our body in poor alignment. Therefore, improved motor fitness will maximise both the safety and effectiveness of our performance.

## How do we improve our motor fitness?

Managing our body weight, manoeuvring our centre of gravity, co-ordinating our body move-

ments, moving at different speeds, in different directions and at different intensities, will all in the long term contribute to improving our motor fitness. If we want to improve our motor fitness, we must specifically and repeatedly train the aspect we wish to improve. If we want to perform a quick, co-ordinated sequence of movements, then we need to perform the specific movements that make up that sequence. However, we may need to train ourselves to develop the necessary skills, which in this example are speed and co-ordination. Therefore, we should break down the sequence into smaller component parts and perform each component in isolation and at a slower pace. By progressively linking one component to another, and moving at a quicker pace, we will, in time, develop the necessary skills to perform the whole sequence at the appropriate speed. We will, therefore, have improved our motor fitness.

Alternatively, if we then wish to learn to walk the tightrope, we need to develop different skills in a different way. Balance will be a very important skill to develop for this activity. Performing our co-ordinated sequence of movements will not assist our balance on the tightrope. Training to improve our motor fitness must therefore specifically relate to the activities we need or want to perform.

We must ensure that we are not deterred if we cannot initially do something. In time, we can all learn the necessary skills to perform any activity. The key is to break down the skill, and allow ourselves the time to develop it slowly. A good teacher will break down the skill for us, and encourage us as we practise and develop.

## How can exercising in water improve our motor fitness?

When we exercise in water we need to learn and develop many different skills. Each of the properties of water will have their individual effect on our body; the extent to which they affect our movements being primarily dependent on our body type, body composition, and distribution of body fat. It is essential that we learn how to manipulate the water to optimise the training benefits we receive. We will need to learn new skills to maintain and regain balance; new skills to manage our centre of buoyancy and to create movement or prevent unwanted movement; and new skills to maintain flotation. The development of these specific skills (propulsive movements, as described in Chapter 1) will provide the greatest improvements to our balance and core stability. Propulsive movements, used effectively, will enhance our performance throughout the whole water-based training programme. They automatically provide a challenge to co-ordination and will maximise the effectiveness of our water-based training and optimise the benefits we receive. They can also be used to assist moving at greater speeds and lifting the body weight out of the water. These are explosive movements that bring further challenge to other components of motor fitness (speed and power).

---

### NEED TO KNOW

Improving motor fitness in a water-based session:

- Speed – perform specific movements at a faster rate.
- Power – use explosive movements that lift the body out of the water.
- Co-ordination – use propulsive movements to assist travel.
- Balance – buoyancy will challenge balance throughout the session, making demands on core stability to maintain upright posture.
- Reaction time and agility – changing and varying the direction of movement sequences will challenge agility and reaction time.

---

## Summary of the benefits of physical fitness

By performing the appropriate types of activity, we can improve each component of physical fitness. Our heart, lungs and circulatory system will become more efficient, allowing us to perform activities for a longer period of time, and without becoming excessively breathless. Our muscles will become stronger, giving us a more toned appearance and improving our posture. Our joints will become more flexible and allow us to move with greater ease. We will move more efficiently and with better control. By improving our physical fitness we are making endless contributions to enhancing our quality of life and maintaining independence.

However, more importantly, by developing our physical fitness we are making a massive contribution to improving our overall health. Being physically fit will keep our heart healthy and decrease the risk of coronary heart disease. It will also keep our bones and joints healthy, preventing the onset of osteoporosis, and allowing us to maintain a fuller range of motion. It will keep our muscles strong, providing greater support to our skeleton and maintain/improve posture. Moving the joints regularly helps to maintain range of motion and can also be used to manage arthritis. Being physically fit can also help us to maintain a healthy body composition/weight, reducing any additional stress on the joints from carrying excess weight. Ultimately, we should potentially live a longer and fuller life!

## What is total fitness?

Health or total fitness requires us to be socially, mentally, emotionally, nutritionally, spiritually and medically fit, as well as physically fit. Our level of physical fitness will affect our overall health or total fitness. However, total fitness requires more than just taking part in regular physical activity. It demands we pay attention to our lifestyle, our diet, our stress levels, our emotions, our ability to communicate, and recognise sometimes we need quite simply to relax and recuperate. Water-based exercise can provide an appropriate medium for developing the components of total fitness.

## What is social fitness?

Social fitness involves interaction and communication. If we improve our physical fitness, we are making ourselves physically more able to participate in a greater range of social activities, sporting and recreational. As a consequence, we can potentially improve our social fitness.

## How can exercising in water improve our social fitness?

Water-based exercising appears to be particularly effective for improving our social fitness. It enhances communication and potentially promotes the development of friendships between a wider range of participants. This may be due to a variety of reasons. Firstly, many aqua sessions include the use of themed, fun music and choreography patterns that require greater interaction between class members. This can include partner or group work that involves moving in different shapes and patterns across the pool. Indeed, the interaction created from using these patterns requires those participating to communicate more actively with each other. It will also allow for the development of a less competitive and more fun environment, which in turn enables participants to relax and enjoy the session much more. However, such methods need not be exclusive to exercise in water: they

just tend to be. Indeed, the majority of land-based exercise classes appear to be much more serious. This is not saying that exercise in water should not be taken seriously, nor that land-based exercise sessions are no fun. From experience, they are just different!

However, perhaps the most important contributory factor to the increased communication in water-based exercise programmes is that our physical appearance and exercise performance are shielded by the water. It is possibly the way we look, and the way we perform, which potentially create the greatest barriers to our communication with others. Therefore, it could be suggested that water-based workouts can help to reduce these barriers and promote more effective communication and interaction between participants.

On land, most activities have us surrounded by mirrors, which require us to be constantly observing our appearance and performance. Mirrors are useful for assisting with the development of correct technique. However, they may increase feelings of self-consciousness about body shape and size, and physical movements. In addition, when we exercise on land our body and movements are totally visible to all those around us. If we are conscious about being out of shape or unco-ordinated, this can potentially make us feel more awkward and embarrassed. It may also cause us to compare ourselves with those around us. This can potentially create greater competition, and lower our self-esteem if we perceive ourselves to be failing. In the long term it may decrease our adherence to a programme of exercise, which may further increase feelings of failure and further lowering of self-esteem.

In water, though, participants who are conscious about the size and shape of their body, and participants who are less co-ordinated, are less noticeable. They will potentially feel more relaxed and temporarily lose their inhibitions.

This can promote greater concentration on the task in hand and assist with their improved performance. As a consequence, they may receive greater physical benefits from the programme. If they adhere to the programme, they will potentially improve their body shape and co-ordination, ultimately providing a positive long-term effect on self-confidence, self-esteem and psychological well-being.

## What is mental and emotional fitness?

Mental and emotional fitness refers to our psychological well-being. The pressures of daily life can have a negative effect on our mental and emotional fitness, causing us to feel tired and stressed. When we feel stressed, we stimulate the release of hormones (adrenaline, noradrenaline and cortisol) that prepare us for fight, flight or freeze. As a consequence, we release sugars into the blood stream to provide energy for the necessary physical action (run or fight). However, all too often we do not take action (fight or flight), but instead stew on our problems. This has a negative effect on our health because sugars are released which can potentially contribute to atherosclerosis (furring up of the artery walls). Stress is therefore a contributory factor to a number of minor and major diseases. These include high blood pressure, coronary heart disease, irritable bowel syndrome and anxiety. It is therefore wise to take some precautionary measures to reduce our stress levels.

## How will exercise improve our mental and emotional fitness?

Regular exercise can assist with effective stress management. The physical exertion necessary to perform exercises provides us with a way of releasing pressures and taking our minds off the stress we incur in our daily life. When we take part in aerobic exercise, we increase the circulation of endorphins, a hormone that gives us an enhanced feeling of well-being. This feeling can last for much longer than the duration of the actual exercise session. Additionally, the long-term improvements to our body shape and physical appearance can enhance self-esteem, self-image and self-confidence. If we feel confident about ourselves we will act confidently. This can potentially have a tremendous effect on our psychological well-being.

## How can exercising in water improve mental and emotional fitness?

Water is a special environment. Relaxing in a hot bath or Jacuzzi has a marvellous effect on relaxing the mind and the muscles. Exercising in water may provide similar relaxing and therapeutic effects. The reduced effects of the gravitational pull will automatically reduce some of the physical stress on the body. The increased effects of buoyancy will create flotation of the limbs, allowing the muscles to relax slightly. It will also support the weight of the body, decreasing the compression of the joints and allowing them to move more freely and with greater ease. The hydrostatic pressure exerted against the body will promote the circulation of a greater volume of blood and assist with removal of waste products that potentially may contribute to physical tension. In addition, the combined effects of hydrostatic pressure and the turbulence of the water against our bodies can provide a massaging effect. This will potentially decrease both physical and mental tension, promoting relaxation of the muscles and mind.

There is also some evidence that immersion in water will reduce the activity of the sympathetic nervous system, which is most active during times of stress when we are preparing to fight or flight (Hall, 1994).

## NEED TO KNOW

- The **sympathetic branch** of the nervous system **speeds up** physiological processes and is very active when the body is under stress.
- The **parasympathetic branch** of the nervous system **slows down** physiological processes.
- Remember: A **para**chute (parasympathetic) **slows down** descent from a plane.

Exercising in water can provide a stimulating and invigorating effect on the body in an environment, which reduces tension and physical stress. However, it is worth noting that participants who are less confident in water may not experience quite the same levels of relaxation as a confident participant! Some participants will wear armbands or life jackets to manage the fear of falling and going under water.

Another way of assisting relaxation can be to use specific relaxation exercises (see Chapter 7) performed at the end of the session. These can be the perfect way to finish if the pool is sufficiently warm. If the pool is cold, they may serve to irritate and create further stress!

## What is nutritional fitness?

Nutritional fitness requires us to eat a balanced diet. The foods we eat will affect how much energy we have. They will also affect our health and well-being. It is worth remembering that there are no bad foods, just poor diets. It is therefore essential that we eat a balanced diet from the main food groups. We should also ensure that the quantity of food we consume is appropriate to meet our requirements.

## How can exercising in water improve nutritional fitness?

Taking part in regular physical activity can make us more aware of the food we eat and more conscious of our diet. There are many textbooks devoted to this area of total fitness, some of which are listed at the end of this book. This text only suggests some general rules for improving our diet.

- Eat less saturated fat. Too much will increase the risk of high cholesterol and increase furring of the artery walls.
- Eat less sugar. Too much will cause tooth decay and promote the risk of adult onset diabetes.
- Eat less salt. Too much will potentially elevate blood pressure.
- Eat more complex carbohydrates. Too little will lower our energy levels.
- Eat sufficient fibre. Too little will potentially cause constipation and other bowel disorders.
- Eat more fruit and vegetables. Five portions per day minimum to ensure adequate vitamin and mineral intake. This can be easily achieved by individuals with a sweet tooth by eating fruit based desserts such as fresh fruit salad or crumbles.
- Eat a sufficient calorie intake. Too few calories will slow down our metabolism and make us feel lethargic, too many will make us put on weight and will be stored as body fat.
- Drink more water. Too little fluid will cause dehydration, potential heat stroke and place an unnecessary stress on the heart.

- Eat when you feel hungry.
- Stop eating when you feel full.

After any water-based activity the appetite is increased due to the energy and calories expended throughout the workout. The best time to replenish our glycogen stores (stored carbohydrate that we need for energy) is within two hours of activity. However, because many of us use exercise to assist with our weight management, it is worthwhile preparing a healthy and nutritional snack to eat after our activity. This will possibly reduce the temptation for us to purchase and consume a less nutritional snack. If we can plan our exercise programme, we can also plan our diet.

## What is medical fitness?

Medical fitness is our state of health and well-being. It requires our body to be in an optimal working order, that is, not injured or ill. Improvements in all the components of physical fitness contribute massively to this aspect of our total fitness.

## How can exercise improve medical fitness?

Regular activity and keeping physically fit can reduce the risk of many medical problems. These include high blood pressure, coronary heart disease, osteoporosis, obesity, diabetes and stress-related illnesses. In addition, regular exercise and our improved fitness can encourage us to eat more healthily, manage stress more effectively, and maintain a healthy body composition. It will also provide a substitute for our less beneficial social activities. This, in turn, may help us to cut down or remove habits that have an adverse effect on our health, such as smoking, drinking excessive alcohol, or eating too much of the less nutritious foods.

Physical activity is also recommended as part of the treatment plan and management for a number of health issues and conditions. These are discussed further in *GP Referral Schemes* (Lawrence & Barnett, 2006).

## How can exercising in water improve medical fitness?

Exercise in water provides a unique support to the body. The body is placed under far less stress while it is exercising. It is therefore potentially a safer and more comfortable alternative form of physical training for the overweight, pregnant, senior, injured, or physically less able participant. Indeed, many land-based exercise programmes may be considered controversial for some of these members of the population. Alternatively, water-based activities are appropriate for virtually everyone. Water-based exercise programmes can therefore potentially enable a larger range of the population to make improvements to their physical fitness and overall well-being. Some of these people would not be able to achieve these improvements in any other way.

A well-structured water-based exercise programme has the potential to bring about all the necessary improvements to physical and total fitness, in a far less stressful environment. However, exercise in water cannot be claimed to be a panacea for all ills. Moreover, it is just one method of promoting physical activity and improving total fitness. The key issue is that for some of the population it is the only form of physical activity they can participate in safely and effectively.

The use of water-based programmes for specific medical conditions is discussed in *GP Referral Schemes* (Lawrence & Barnett, 2006).

## Spiritual fitness

Spiritual fitness is hard to define specifically. For some it relates to religious beliefs and for others it relates to their sense of self. For this author, it embraces the humanistic notion of being all that we can be, knowing and being content with the person we are. The type of person we become and the choices we make can be influenced by belief systems, attitudes and values passed down through our family system, educational system, society and cultural systems, and religious systems. Each of these can impact our own belief systems, our mental outlook (how we view our self and our life), our emotional management (how we respond to our own feelings and emotions, and how we respond to the feelings and emotions of others); our attitude to physical activity (our activity levels and whether we look at exercise as a pleasure or an inconvenience), our eating behaviour (the type of food we eat and size of our plate), our lifestyle choices (transport, smoking, alcohol, hobbies), and our social relationships (how we relate to others, prejudices etc).

Achieving physical fitness can lead us to developing other aspects of our self and improving our overall health (nutritional and medical etc), which in turn can enhance the way in which we relate to ourselves, others and our community. Finding the inner power to make changes to ourselves (getting fitter, eating well, making friends etc) to improve our own world is refreshing and empowering for our 'spirit'. Water, movement, music and dance all create space to focus on the self and engage with the spirit or the fun loving and free aspect inside ourselves.

## SUMMARY OF THE BENEFITS OF EXERCISING IN WATER

Exercising in water will potentially:
- improve all components of physical fitness
- assist with weight management
- promote social interaction
- encourage a healthier lifestyle
- provide a marvellous therapeutic and relaxing effect
- assist with stress management
- assist with the management and prevention of some medical conditions
- enhance feelings of well-being
- improve overall health
- help us to achieve our full potential.

# SHORT ANSWER REVISION QUESTIONS

1. Name the body systems improved by:
   (a) training cardiovascular fitness
   (b) muscular strength and endurance training
   (c) flexibility training.

2. Describe the difference between:
   (a) static and dynamic stretching
   (b) muscular strength and endurance.

3. Describe the terms: prime mover, antagonist and fixator.

4. Describe the terms: concentric, eccentric and static.

5. Name the waste product of the glycogen energy system.

6. State **TWO** benefits of:
   (a) cardiovascular training
   (b) MSE training
   (c) flexibility training.

7. Name the **THREE** main energy systems.

8. Describe the difference between aerobic and anaerobic.

9. Give **ONE** example of an activity that would use the:
   (a) aerobic energy system
   (b) glycogen/lactic acid energy system
   (c) creatine phosphate energy system.

10. State the American College of Sports Medicine (ACSM, 2006) FITT (frequency, intensity, time and type) training guidelines for improving:
    (a) muscular fitness
    (b) improving flexibility
    (c) CV fitness.

11. Describe social fitness.

12. Describe mental and emotional fitness.

13. List **SIX** ways exercise in water (aqua) may contribute to improving total fitness/health.

# HEALTH AND SAFETY FOR PLANNING A WATER-BASED EXERCISE PROGRAMME

**PART TWO**

2

# GATHERING INFORMATION FROM THE TARGET GROUP

3

## OBJECTIVES

By the end of this chapter the reader will be able to:

- Identify the range of participants who may attend a water-based exercise session
- Recognise different methods for collecting and gathering information from participants in relation to their health and fitness status
- Identify some advantages and disadvantages of using different methods of screening.

## Who can benefit from water-based training?

The answer to this is quite simple: everybody can benefit from water-based exercising. Water possesses resistive properties that can be manipulated, if desired, to provide an intense and physically challenging workout for the cardio-vascular and muscular systems. It is therefore an effective training environment for those who work out regularly and for sportspeople. Water also possesses unique supportive properties and consequently it is potentially a far less stressful training environment than land. It is therefore an ideal training medium for populations with more specialist needs and requirements.

Water-based exercise programmes attract a wide range of the population. A selection of those who may attend are outlined in table 3.1.

| Table 3.1 | Populations who may attend water-based training programmes |
|---|---|

- Confident swimmers, less confident swimmers and non-swimmers
- The fit and the unfit
- Different genders (male and female)
- Different body shapes and sizes
- Different age groups (adults, children, teenagers, seniors)
- Athletes and sportspeople
- Specialist groups (ante- and post-natal, seniors, children)
- Persons with other specialist requirements (joint problems, medical problems).

# Is it safe for anyone to start exercising in water?

Most people can be accommodated quite safely in a water-based exercise session. However, there are some participants who will need to obtain permission from their doctor before embarking on any programme of physical activity. This is to ensure that the exercise programme will be appropriate to their needs and that they will not be placing their well-being at risk by participating in the session. It is wise to check with a doctor, prior to taking part in any physical activity, if an individual answers yes to any of the conditions outlined in table 3.2.

Identifying the fitness goals and current health state of individuals is the first step to designing an appropriate water-based training programme. It is also necessary to take into account the working environment. It is ineffective to design a programme without making such considerations.

The programme may be potentially unsafe if it is performed in an inappropriate environment without specific adaptations being made.

# How can the teacher get this information from their target group?

There are three methods of gaining information from and about the target group.
- Visual (observing gender, age, body shape and size)
- Verbal (things you need to ask and be told by the participant)
- Written (questions – Physical Activity Readiness Questionnaire – PAR-Q).

A few of the advantages and disadvantages of the different screening methods are identified in table 3.3 on page 60.

| Table 3.2 | Health screening checks |
| --- | --- |

Check with a doctor and seek their consent prior to commencing any physical activity if you:
- have high blood pressure, heart disease or cardiovascular or respiratory problems
- have suffered from chest pains, especially if associated with light activity requiring minimal effort
- are prone to headaches, fainting or dizziness
- are pregnant or have recently been pregnant
- have, or are recovering from, a joint problem or injury that may be aggravated by physical activity
- are taking medication or have any other medical condition
- have recently been ill
- are unused to exercise and over 35 years of age
- have breathing problems such as asthma (specific to water)
- have skin infections or open wounds (specific to water).

| Table 3.3 | Advantages and disadvantages of different methods of screening | |
|---|---|---|
| Method of screening | Advantages | Disadvantages |
| Visual | • Quick<br>• Can identify more personal issues (obesity) without having to ask questions that may be embarrassing<br>• Can identify if individuals are wearing correct attire | • Cannot identify all medical ailments visually |
| Verbal | • Response is immediate<br>• Information is up to date<br>• Personal contact<br>• Can probe and seek further information if necessary<br>• Can highlight the importance of receiving the information<br>• Can clarify and respond to any questions asked | • Participants may be unwilling to provide personal information.<br>• Responses may not be totally truthful<br>• There is no written record or proof of what has been asked, nor the response provided<br>• Information provided may be forgotten<br>• Time-consuming, since only one person can be spoken to at a time<br>• Confidentiality – information should be obtained in private |
| Written | • Permanent record of questions asked and responses provided<br>• If the questionnaire used provides a yes or no response, concerns can be identified relatively quickly<br>• Can screen more than one person at a time | • Circumstances change, therefore written screening should be updated regularly<br>• Screening forms need to be stored in a secure place and remain confidential<br>• Questionnaires need to be worded carefully to obtain the accurate response<br>• Information requested needs to encourage a concise response (yes/no). Wordy responses may be difficult to interpret and will take longer to read<br>• Reading the responses to questionnaires is time-consuming |

## SHORT ANSWER REVISION QUESTIONS

1. List **FOUR** different types of client who may attend a water-based training session.

2. Give **TWO** reasons why it is essential to gather information from the target group regarding their readiness to exercise.

3. State **ONE** advantage and **ONE** disadvantage of visual screening.

4. State **ONE** advantage and **ONE** disadvantage of verbal screening.

5. State **ONE** advantage and **ONE** disadvantage of written screening.

6. Give **TWO** instances when you may advise an individual to seek medical advice before participating in an exercise in water session.

# POOL SAFETY AND ADAPTING TO WORK IN THE POOL ENVIRONMENT

4

## OBJECTIVES

By the end of this chapter the reader will be able to:

- Identify some of the similarities and differences between various pool training environments
- Recognise a range of safety considerations that are necessary prior to planning a safe and effective water-based session
- Describe different methods of adapting session content and structure to work in different pool environments (pool shapes, water depths, location, pool and poolside design etc).

## How do pools differ?

Water-based exercise programmes can take place in a variety of pool locations. The majority of pool activities in the United Kingdom tend to be indoors. However, in warmer climates and where outdoor pools are accessible, they can take place in the open air. Each pool environment will have its own structural peculiarities. A specific programme of activities may work effectively and be totally suitable for one pool location, yet may be totally ineffective and unsuitable for another. Recognising the limitations of certain pool environments will help to identify some appropriate strategies for maximising the safety and effectiveness of the water-based exercise session.

Each of these factors will have an effect on the programme design, the number of participants that can safely participate, and the working practice of the instructor/teacher. They will therefore need to be considered in the planning of the programme. Any pre-prepared programmes would need to be adapted to accommodate the specific environmental differences, to ensure that they adhere to the approved code of practice for health and safety.

This chapter identifies some of the necessary safety considerations for working in different pool environments. It also provides practical guidelines for adapting session content and structure when working in different pools.

### NEED TO KNOW

The primary differences between pools include:

- water depth
- shape and size of the pool
- water level
- pool fixtures
- pool surface
- space and surface of poolside
- pool temperature
- working rules and regulations – number of lifeguards etc.

# What is the ideal water depth?

The majority of water-based exercises require a water depth between waist and chest level for their safe and effective performance. However, the participants who take part in water-based exercise sessions are all different. They will be of different heights, shapes, body compositions, fitness levels, and may have varying levels of skill and confidence in the water. Therefore, there is no one water depth or pool design that can be advocated as most appropriate.

In an ideal world, participants could alter their depth at different times throughout the programme, enabling them to select a depth of water that suited their own requirements and the requirements of the exercise. However, in reality this is virtually impossible, and very difficult to manage for an instructor who is dealing with large groups of people. It is much easier for an instructor to manage appropriate alterations of water depth when personally training a client in a private pool or, indeed, during their own training sessions.

# What safety considerations should be made when working in a children's teaching pool?

Teaching pools are very shallow. They provide less support to body weight due to increased effects of gravity when exercising in shallow water. Jumping, jogging and explosive movements are less appropriate in these pools because the impact forces received are not reduced so effectively. It is therefore necessary to select exercises that reduce the impact forces on the body to maximise safety, and reduce stress on the weight-bearing joints.

A common alternative is to use the arms out of the water, but this is not necessarily safer or more effective because the momentum created by the speed of these movements against the force of gravity may potentially cause movements to be uncontrolled, placing unnecessary stress on the upper body muscles and joints. In addition, a considerable amount of high arm work out of the water may potentially elevate blood pressure. But, more importantly, the use of arms out of the water is less effective. Working the arms without the resistance of the water will make fewer demands on the larger muscles of the back and chest due to the change of muscular contraction when working against gravity. Instead, the smaller muscles of the shoulder (the deltoids) will tend to be responsible for assisting the performance for most of these exercises. The use of the smaller muscles, combined with a reduced resistance, will potentially lower the volume of oxygen required to perform the exercise, reducing both cardiovascular and muscular endurance benefits. So, other ways of challenging the cardiovascular and muscular endurance components of fitness will need to be found.

## NEED TO KNOW

- In a children's teaching pool the water depth is considerably lower/more shallow.
- In shallow water, the effects of gravity are higher than in deeper water. This means that any higher impact exercise will still be affected by the gravitational force (approximately 50 per cent).

# What types of activities are appropriate for a teaching pool session?

A potentially safer and more effective alternative form of training for shallow water is to alternate arm exercises under the water with lower impact travelling movements for the lower body. Kneeling or squatting in the water to perform large-range arm movements will once again utilise the muscles of the chest and back. However, we must consider the discomfort that may be caused by squatting or kneeling continuously. Alternating the use of the upper body moves under the water with leg-biased travelling movements through the water, such as wading and side squatting, should alleviate any discomfort. In addition, we must consider how to vary stress on the upper body joints even in this position. Varying the direction of the arm movements under the water will encourage the work of different muscle groups and will consequently alter the stress placed on the upper body joints. Varying the direction of travelling movements will sufficiently alter any stress placed on the lower body. Ultimately, a movement sequence combining a variety of the movements described above should sufficiently alter the stress on the body. It will also be effective, provided that the intensity of movements is sufficient to create challenge.

An alternative, and relatively new approach, to water-based exercising – water walking – would be very effective. Walking in different directions around the pool, using different stride lengths, moving at different speeds, will create variety and intensity in this type of programme. Indeed, this type of session could complement the range of other water-based programmes that can be safely delivered in a teaching pool.

Some muscular strength and endurance exercises may be less effective. If the hip is out of the water, there will be less resistance to standing side leg raises at the poolside. The upper body will also cool down quicker if it is out of the water for too long. Therefore, alternative positions will need to be found to maximise the effort from participants, and to maintain a comfortable temperature. It is often safer and more effective to combine the cardiovascular and muscular strength and endurance activities in this type of pool, so a circuit training approach, where exercises training each component are alternated, can work quite well in a teaching pool.

Some stretch positions may also be less safe, and possibly no longer achievable. The hamstring stretch, where the leg is lifted to the surface of the water, may be less effective due to the smaller range of motion achieved. This is of course dependent on the flexibility of the individual. However, movement of the leg out of the water will increase the effects of gravity. This may reduce the ability of the opposing muscle, the quadriceps, to relax, making the stretch potentially more active. In addition, if the arm is used to assist the stretch and balance is lost, the muscle may potentially exceed its range of motion. This will create a ballistic movement that may potentially cause damage or tearing of the muscle. Therefore, stretch positions will also need to be adapted in this type of pool, if they are to be performed safely.

One advantage of working in a teaching pool is that the water temperature is generally high. This means that a longer duration can be set aside for stretching and relaxation exercises, providing the opportunity to design a specific stretch and relaxation water programme. Indeed, in most pools this type of programme would be totally unsuitable because the normal working temperatures require high levels of pulse-raising to be maintained throughout the session, which is not totally conducive to the aims of the programme. However, even in a warmer pool it may still be necessary to intersperse a reasonable number of

## SUMMARY OF ADAPTATIONS FOR WORKING IN A TEACHING POOL

- Decrease the amount of jumping and explosive moves
- Increase travelling movements through the water and the use of arm work under the water to create effective cardiovascular training
- Use alternative positions for muscular strength and endurance work to maximise resistance of water
- Alternate cardiovascular and muscular strength and endurance exercises
- Adapt stretch positions to maximise the support of buoyancy
- Spend longer on stretching and relaxation components due to warmer water and air temperature.

### Alternative approaches to programme structure

- Circuit training for a combined cardiovascular, muscular strength and endurance workout
- Water walking for cardiovascular training
- Stretch and relax for a unique approach to flexibility improvement and stress management
- Stretch and tone for a combined muscular strength, muscular endurance and flexibility workout.

range of motion stretches and mobility exercises throughout such programmes to maintain an appropriate body temperature.

It would appear that a teaching pool is not the most ideal environment for water-based exercising. This is true to some extent, but they are quite frequently the only pool space accessible. Therefore, it is essential that the exercises and session structure are adapted to maximise the safety and effectiveness of the programme. It is preferable to adapt and provide another opportunity for promoting fitness and health, than to limit the opportunities available.

## What safety considerations should be noted when working in a pool with a constant water depth?

Some of the more recreational pools have a constant depth of water. The depth can vary from pool to pool, although most will allow a person of average height to stand with the water somewhere between waist and chest depth. In many ways, a constant depth can provide many advantages. There is no danger of suddenly moving out of your depth, and modifications to session structure and exercise selection are minimal in comparison to other pool depth variations. However, a key disadvantage is that if you are below the average height, you may not be able to participate without the use of a buoyancy aid.

## What types of activities are appropriate for working in a pool with a constant water depth?

Realistically, most exercises are appropriate, although it would obviously not be possible to programme a deep-water session! In addition, while the majority of the population should be able to perform most exercises relatively safely in this type of pool, shorter people may be totally excluded, unless they use buoyancy aids to keep them afloat. If this is necessary for them to take part, then further consideration will need to be given to the speed at which they can move, and the extra effort they will need to exert to keep pace with other participants in a group session. Exercises will therefore need to be individually modified, so that they are able to achieve the desired training response.

Alternatively, very tall people may not be provided with sufficient support (buoyancy) to perform a large proportion of jumping or explosive movements. This is dependent on both the depth of water and the height of the person. Therefore, it will be necessary to adapt some exercises to accommodate these individuals, and maximise the safety and effectiveness of the programme for them.

A key disadvantage of working in these pools is that they allow no alteration of water depth. Varying the depth of water can assist those with more buoyant body types and those less confident in water, with their performance of some exercises. A sound working knowledge of the properties of water, discussed earlier, should be sufficient to identify the various adaptations that can be made to suit these individuals, as and when necessary. Ultimately, a constant depth of water will allow for the majority of people to take part, with relatively fewer adaptations to the exercises selected and structure of the session.

## NEED TO KNOW

- When working in pools with a constant water depth (same depth), adaptations will need to be given to accommodate people who are different heights (taller and shorter).
- Taller people may need to perform less explosive movements to reduce the effects of gravity and impact on their joints.

## SUMMARY OF ADAPTATIONS FOR WORKING IN A CONSTANT WATER DEPTH

- Provide flotation equipment for shorter participants and those less confident in water, if necessary. Allow them to work at a slower pace if such equipment is used
- Provide adaptations to jumping and explosive work for very tall people to reduce impact
- Aim to select exercises which can be comfortably performed by different people regardless of the water depth. For example, replace standing poolside leg raises with suspended poolside scissor legs
- Be ready to adapt the intensity of any exercise by alternative means. Decreasing or increasing the range of motion, lengthening or shortening levers, decreasing or increasing speed, etc. may compensate for the lack of opportunity to adapt water depth to suit certain individual requirements.

### Alternative approaches to programme structure
- Circuit training for a combined cardiovascular and muscular strength and endurance workout.
- Step training for cardiovascular training
- Water walking programmes.

## What safety considerations should be noted when working in a pool with a changing water depth?

All pools should clearly indicate the depth of water at different distances. However, the changes of water depth can vary from a gradual sloping descent to a fairly sudden drop. A key disadvantage of working in a pool where the depth changes suddenly is that participants can easily move out of their depth. Therefore, when a group session is planned it is wise to rope off the point where the depth changes suddenly.

It is also essential that participants are orientated to the changes of water depth at the start of the session. This can be achieved practically, by allowing them to enter the pool and encouraging them to walk around carefully to explore the water depth. However, further verbal reminders will need to be reinforced throughout the session, when their concentration becomes more focused on their workout. These initial precautionary measures can ensure participants stay in a safe and comfortable depth of water at all times.

A further precaution is to advise non-swimmers' or those less confident in water, to position themselves well away from where the depth changes suddenly, and ideally in slightly shallower water closer to the poolside. However, while they should be close enough for the instructor to provide assistance, they should not be so close that their movements will be endangered by the poolside. A final precaution is to make their whereabouts known to a lifeguard, who can keep a watchful eye throughout the session.

## What types of activities are appropriate for working in a pool with a changing water depth?

This will depend on whether the change of depth is sudden or sloping. The types of activities for sloping floors are discussed in the next paragraph. Alternatively, for pools with a constant and then sudden change of depth, it is perhaps not advisable to perform movements towards where the depth changes. However, if the area is roped off then they may be appropriate. Other than this, the advice regarding exercise selection for working in a constant pool depth is all that will need to be considered.

### NEED TO KNOW

- Rope off areas where water depth changes suddenly to ensure people do not move out of their depth in the session.

## What safety considerations should be noted when working in a pool with a sloping floor?

A sloping pool floor can encourage accidental movement out of the appropriate water depth. Travelling movements, and movements creating a lot of turbulence, are most likely to cause the biggest problems. The safety precautions previously identified for pools with changing water depths are applicable to this type of pool.

## What types of activities are appropriate for working in a pool with a sloping floor?

Further precautions can be taken by designing movements that travel across the direction of the slope, rather than towards it. Participants who are confident in water may well enjoy and be entertained by moving towards the slope and out of their depth. However, those who are less confident will be fearful and will find little enjoyment in such movements. Alternatively, they may well be entertained by seeing someone who is confident in water quite happily disappear and re-appear from the surface of the water. Therefore these movement patterns can be included, providing the non-swimmers and those less confident are initially positioned in much shallower water.

Alternatively, travelling towards the shallower water first may be another appropriate precautionary measure, though care should be taken if a stationary jumping movement precedes the travel. In shallow water, the impact forces are much higher, and jumping movements are more stressful. At least in deep water the exercise can be performed in a suspended state, and remain less stressful to the joints.

Another key problem associated with working on an uneven surface is the potential misalignment of correct posture. It is not ideal to have either the toes or heels positioned higher than the other. This can create an unnatural forward or backward lean. Additionally, the body will be equally unbalanced if one leg is positioned higher than the other. The constant performance of exercises from the same starting position and in the same direction will exaggerate these problems. This could potentially lead to the creation of muscle imbalance and the possible risk of injury.

The degree of muscular imbalance that is created will to some extent be dependent on the gradient of the slope. A mildly sloping pool can still be appropriate for a water-based exercise session. However, the session will need to be adapted to ensure there are sufficient variations of direction, starting position, footstrike and landing position. Such modifications will ensure that some attempt is made to maintain muscle balance. A circuit training class structure is often the most appropriate session for this type of pool. Circuit training sessions generally promote plenty of movement around the pool, and allow a variety of exercise positions to be performed. A further advantage is that they frequently alternate jumping and jogging activities for the cardiovascular system, with muscular strength and endurance exercises at the poolside. This will create further variation of stress to the body.

Pools with excessively sloping bottoms are not appropriate for shallow water-based training sessions. They will further exaggerate the problems associated with postural alignment, and will increase the likelihood of moving out of a comfortable depth. However, for deep-water training programmes they are perfectly suitable. Ultimately, it is much more beneficial to design a new deep-water session, rather than lose an opportunity to promote exercise and fitness.

## What safety considerations should be noted when working in a pool where the depth can be altered mechanically?

Some centres provide access to a pool where the floor is moveable. The key safety considerations are that the pool is free of exercisers when the floor is altered, and that participants take care not to catch their feet where the pool floor meets the poolside.

## SUMMARY OF ADAPTATIONS FOR WORKING IN A POOL WITH A CHANGING DEPTH AND/OR SLOPING FLOOR

- Rope off the area where water depth changes suddenly
- Encourage participants to familiarise themselves with sudden depth changes
- Advise non-swimmers to exercise close to the poolside and in shallower water depths
- Notify the lifeguard of the whereabouts of non-swimmers
- Travel across sloping floors to avoid movement out of depth
- Only travel towards the slope if there is sufficient space, or if participants closer to the deeper water are confident and willing to move slightly out of their depth when performing travelling movements
- Vary the starting position and direction of travel for different exercises to alter the mechanical stress and avoid a potential muscle imbalance that can be created by working on a pool with a sloping floor
- Use the pool for deep-water programmes if the slope is excessive.

**Alternative approaches to programme structure**
- Circuit training for a combined cardiovascular and muscular strength and endurance workout
- Water walking for cardiovascular training
- Deep-water training.

## What types of activities are appropriate for working in a pool where the depth can be altered mechanically?

The depth of these pools can be altered to suit the activity. They can be made deeper for diving, synchronised swimming and deep-water programmes, or shallower for a variety of other water-based exercise programmes. It is because the depth is variable that a variety of participants can be accommodated and a variety of exercises can be performed. A mild slope of the pool floor will allow persons of varying heights to participate and exercise at an appropriate depth. It will also allow them to vary their depth to suit the activity or their different requirements. The advantage is that it is unlikely that any participant will move totally out of

their depth when working in these pools, unless of course the slope is too extreme, in which case it is probably not appropriate to use. However, if the pool floor is sloped, then the safety considerations that apply to the sloping pool are equally applicable, and need to be accommodated. Alternatively, if the pool floor is set at a constant depth, then the safety considerations and adaptations for working in this type of pool are necessary.

## What safety considerations should be noted when working in a hydrotherapy pool?

Hydrotherapy pools are heated to a slightly higher temperature than pools used for recreational activities. This is to allow for the treatment of a range of specialist conditions by qualified physiotherapists. However, a contraindication of working in hotter hydrotherapy pools is the body's less effective management of heat loss. Even light exercising in a pool with a very high temperature can have adverse effects on the body. It is therefore recommended that those designing programmes that are to be implemented in a hydrotherapy pool should liaise closely with a physiotherapist regarding the necessary further considerations prior to the design and structure of the programme.

## NEED TO KNOW

Exercise intensity would need to be reduced when working in a hydrotherapy pool.

## What types of activities are appropriate for working in a hydrotherapy pool?

Providing the pool temperature is not too high and does not exceed 33°C (92°F), low intensity programmes can be implemented safely and effectively. However, those with specialist medical conditions should only be trained by instructors who are knowledgeable and qualified to deal with their requirements.

For general populations, warming up can consist of predominantly lower intensity mobility movements. Mobility exercises that maximise the support of the water and move slowly through the full range of motion should be sufficient to warm the body and replace the traditional pulse-raising activities used for exercising in cooler pools. In addition, a greater

proportion of static stretches can be used without the body cooling down too much. However, any cardiovascular training should be of a much lower level. Gentle walking exercises and lower intensity moves that are traditionally used for warming the body before the main workout in a cooler pool, can replace more intense activities. Lower intensity muscular strength and endurance activities, which require the body to work more slowly through the full range of motion, should be appropriate. Additionally, there will be less need for movements to maintain body warmth because the exercises themselves should help to maintain a reasonable body temperature. A higher proportion of time can be spent on relaxation and stretching at the end of the session because the body will not cool down so quickly.

An advantage of working in a pool with a relatively warmer temperature is that a higher proportion of static stretches can be used, and greater time can be spent on specific relaxation techniques and much slower range of motion mobility work. It is therefore an ideal environment to implement a specific stretch and relaxation session. Using a combination of full range of motion mobility work, slow moving and static stretches with a higher proportion of specific relaxation exercises can be very therapeutic.

A final use for a hydrotherapy pool is to implement a programme specifically for senior participants, or indeed others with specialist conditions such as rheumatism and arthritis. The warmer water temperatures allow them to move at a necessarily slower and more controlled pace without the fear of cooling down excessively. However, it is essential that any specialist groups are only trained by those who are competent to deal with their requirements, and only after referral from their doctor or physiotherapist.

## SUMMARY OF ADAPTATIONS FOR WORKING IN A HYDROTHERAPY POOL

- Use slow full range of motion mobility work for warming up at a lower intensity
- Use a higher proportion of static stretches
- Any cardiovascular training should be of a much lower intensity and possibly for a shorter duration
- Lower to moderate intensity muscular strength and endurance (toning) work can be performed without the need to include other movements to keep warm
- Ideally spend much more time on mobilising, stretching and relaxation components due to warmer water and air temperature.

### Alternative approaches to programme structure

- Mobilise, stretch and tone for a combined mobility, flexibility and muscular strength and endurance workout
- Mobilise, stretch and relax for a unique approach to flexibility improvement and stress management
- Lower intensity circuit training programmes comprising water walking, and isolated low intensity muscular exercises for a combined cardiovascular and muscular strength and endurance workout
- Specialist seniors' programmes (instructors should be competent and qualified to deal with their specialist requirements)
- Injury rehabilitation programmes (with guidance and referral from a qualified physiotherapist).

## How will the shape and size of a pool affect the session?

Some pools are large and are designed to host a wide variety of water-based activities at the same time. These can include swimming, diving and other family activities and recreation. Some pools are smaller and may be unsuitable for diving, being primarily designed for recreational activities and swimming. In some swimming centres a number of different pools are accessible, each being designed to suit a particular activity. However, very few pools are solely designed for water-based exercise sessions.

The majority of pools tend to be square or rectangular in shape. However, there are some pools that have slightly more peculiar shapes, such as kidney, 'L', oval, and circular. The size of the pool, its shape, and the amount of space providing water at the appropriate depth will clearly restrict the number of participants that can safely take part in the session. It is recommended that even in larger pools where space is generous, class numbers should still be restricted to a maximum of 25–30 participants. This will promote greater safety and help the instructor to manage and observe all participants carefully throughout. If larger class numbers are necessary, there should be appropriately qualified 'spotters' available to assist the instructor. In addition, extra pool lifeguards should be requested. Ideally, if the popularity of a particular session increases, then such demands should be accommodated by expanding the aqua programme and increasing the number and variety of sessions available. This will potentially provide better customer care and improve the service. It will also allow for those with special requirements to attend the most appropriate session to meet their needs, rather than the only session that is available!

The size and shape of the pool, and number of participants exercising, will also potentially place restrictions on the exercises that are selected. Movements which require considerable travel in different directions can only safely and effectively be achieved if there is sufficient space to perform them. It may therefore be necessary to adapt the programme to suit the shape of the pool. If exercising alone in a private pool, you can move around to your heart's content. If you are training a client in a personal or quiet pool, you can also move around quite freely. However, if sharing the pool with other users, you need to ensure that you are sensitive to their spatial requirements, as well as your own. If the session is specifically geared towards a group of participants, then dramatic changes may be necessary.

When space is limited, the aerobic or cardio-vascular component of the workout should comprise a variety of more static exercises such as jogging, jumping and explosive movements. To avoid the workout becoming too intense and too repetitive, it is advisable to combine these leg movements with strong movements of the arms under the water.

The main workout can be designed so that participants work in two circular groups: the outer circle can move in one direction, the inner circle in the other. A combination of jogging and walking in this circular format with occasional stationary exercises using the arms, can be very effective. However, it should be noted that movement in this way can increase eddy currents and turbulence. This will intensify the

workout and make it harder to maintain balance, so care needs to be taken with those less confident in water. Alternatively, equipment can be used to increase the intensity of cardio-vascular exercises and substitute the intensity lost from the reduction of travelling moves.

In some pools there may be limited space available at the poolside for the performance of muscular strength, endurance and stretching exercises. These exercises will therefore need to be performed in the centre of the pool, using propulsive movements to maintain balance. If a sufficient amount of equipment is accessible (floats or tubes), then it can be used to assist balance or intensify the movements of exercises performed mid-pool. This will also add variety to the programme. However, it must be ensured that participants are able to use any equipment safely and effectively.

## How will the shape and size of a pool affect the instructor?

The shape and size of a pool will also affect the different teaching positions accessible by the instructor. A small square or rectangular pool may well allow the instructor to move freely around the poolside. However, larger and wider pools will restrict movement around the pool. In addition, other poolside obstructions such as diving boards, slides and flumes may restrict this even further.

### NEED TO KNOW

The shape and size of the pool will determine the extent by which the instructor can move around the pool and the number of teaching positions/class fronts available.

## SUMMARY OF ADAPTATIONS FOR WORKING IN DIFFERENT SIZE POOLS

- Use spotters to assist in larger pools, when accommodating larger class numbers, or when teaching very mixed ability groups
- Have extra lifeguards available to observe in larger pools and in dealing with larger groups
- Restrict class numbers in smaller pools
- Ideally, expand the centre's aqua programme if classes become popular
- When space is limited, decrease the travelling movements and use more stationary exercises
- When travelling moves have to be limited, alternate the use of arms and legs to alter the stress placed on the joints
- Use mid-pool muscular strength and endurance exercises if there is a lack of space at pool-side. Flotation equipment can be used to assist balance and add variety
- Use mid-pool stretches with propulsive movements to assist balance where necessary
- Instructors/teachers should adapt their coaching position to ensure they can see and be seen at all times.

## How will water level affect the session?

Some pools have a large gap between the water and poolside. Others allow the water to lap over the edge. If the water laps over the poolside, the water will be slightly less turbulent. If the water rebounds against the wall of the pool, the water will be more turbulent. For example, sea water is much more turbulent when it moves against rocks, than when it rolls up the beach.

The greater the turbulence in the water, the greater will be the effort required to maintain balance. Additionally, the resistance from the water to the body movements will also be increased. Therefore, the exercises selected may need to be those that do not create excessive turbulence. It may be necessary to travel less and select

exercise patterns that allow the group to move in a more linear fashion, as opposed to using staggered and random movements, such as some circuit training formats. However, this will be dependent on the fitness of participants, their confidence and skill in the water, and the activity they are performing. In addition, turbulence will be increased if a greater number of bodies are participating, so it may be safer to limit the number of class participants exercising at the same time.

### NEED TO KNOW

There will be greater turbulence and eddy resistance in a pool where the water level is much lower than the pool edge.

## How will water level affect safety when moving on the poolside?

A key disadvantage of having a pool where the water flows over the surface is that the poolside will be more slippery. This will affect the safety of the instructor and lifeguards when moving around the pool. It will also affect the safety of participants as they enter and exit the pool. It is therefore essential that everyone using the poolside is advised to move around with extreme caution.

## How will the fixtures at the pool wall affect the session?

Some pools have gullies, ledges or stainless steel rails at the pool wall. These are useful and can assist with the performance of certain poolside exercises. If the pool is equipped with a gully or bar, then a large variety of exercises can be included at the poolside. The security of pool rails and cleanliness of the gullies should be checked by pool attendants.

It is useful to check the surface of the pool wall. An abrasive pool wall may cause discomfort during the performance of some exercises, and may damage the participants' swimwear. If this is the case, forewarn participants, and ideally provide an alternative for exercises that require contact by the body with the pool wall.

## How will the surface of the pool floor affect the session?

In an ideal world, all the pools we use for our water-based exercising would be non-slippery and non-scratchy. Scratchy pool surfaces will provide better traction and grip, but they are abrasive and unkind to the skin on the feet. They can cause soreness to the feet after only one session. It is advisable to wear some kind of footwear to protect the feet.

Slippery pool surfaces make it difficult to maintain a secure foothold, and make it easier to lose balance. This may be particularly distressing for those with less confidence in water. It may also reduce the intensity of travelling movements. The use of appropriate aquatic footwear may provide some traction, and will help to promote more effective balance. If worn, it may assist with the performance of movements, maximising their effectiveness. It may also promote greater safety by assisting the prevention of misalignment of the joints and subsequent damage to their surrounding tissues. If no footwear is worn, it may be necessary to include fewer travelling movements so that joint alignment and balance can be maintained more easily.

## How will the poolside affect the session?

The majority of poolsides are made of concrete and are usually very slippery. On occasions they are covered with a matting that reduces the slipperiness of their surface. It is advisable for instructors to arrive early to ensure the poolside is dry and free from any unnecessary obstruction or hazard.

The condition of the poolside will affect the safety of participants as they enter or exit the pool. They should therefore be instructed to move with care and, if necessary, be provided with assistance. However, the condition of the poolside will primarily affect the safety of the instructor, and their ability to move around the pool to demonstrate, observe and correct. Be particularly careful when demonstrating exercises or moving around the poolside. Perform far fewer repetitions of intense jumping movements and instead use visual instructions and other verbal cues. Take the lower impact option to the move more frequently to prevent stress to the joints. The use of mini-trampolines and mats on the poolside can be equally hazardous, and it is not easy to demonstrate travelling movements using such devices. The use of supportive trainers will provide some stress relief and support for the joints, though they too can be slippery on the poolside.

Teachers should also be aware of the risk of overusing the voice, which may stress the vocal cords. It is advisable for all teachers to receive appropriate vocal training.

# How will pool and air temperature affect the session?

The temperature of the pool and its effect on water-based activities has been discussed in Chapter 1.

# What are the safety considerations for working in an outdoor pool?

The opportunity to coach in an outdoor pool in a warmer climate may be regarded as the ultimate luxury. However, precautions need to be taken to ensure the instructor and participants are not unnecessarily exposed to the rays of the sun. Exercising when the sun's rays are strongest should be avoided at all costs. All exercisers should use protective suntan lotions, and cover body areas most vulnerable to burning. It is also advisable for participants to wear a long-sleeved, fitted T-shirt under their costume to protect their arms and shoulders from exposure to the sun. In addition, sports caps can be worn to protect the head.

It is essential that the instructor and participants are kept fully hydrated when exercising in warmer temperatures. Plastic water bottles can be kept on the poolside for easy access. It may be necessary to lower the intensity of the workout for those unaccustomed to working out in hotter pool and air temperatures.

In the event of an electrical storm, it is important for safety to leave the outdoor pool. Evacuation will be controlled by the lifeguard at a public pool; in a private or home pool, exercisers are advised to leave the pool immediately.

# What other rules and regulations will affect working practice on the poolside?

The working rules and regulations will vary from one pool venue to another. It is therefore essential that these rules and regulations, as well as the specific peculiarities of the working environment, are identified prior to the design and implementation of any water-based exercise programme. The instructor/teacher should be able to locate and operate:

- the nearest telephone
- fire exits
- fire extinguishers
- rescue and safety equipment
- number of lifeguards
- First Aid kit
- emergency buttons/alarms, etc.

Adherence to an appropriate code of practice will promote safer and effective exercising for all involved.

## How to promote pool hygiene

The maintenance of a clean pool is primarily the responsibility of the centre. Chlorine is used in most pools as a sterilising agent. However, it will fade colour, so anything used in the pool should be rinsed after use in the water to preserve its condition and colour. This includes equipment used throughout the session, and the clothing worn by participants.

The instructor can contribute to appropriate pool hygiene by:

• advising participants to shower and use foot baths before they enter the pool, as well as when they exit
• using footwear exclusively for the poolside
• encouraging participants to tie back long hair
• encouraging attendants to regularly mop and dry the poolside (especially prior to their session)
• checking that chlorine levels are monitored regularly.

## How can entry to and exit from the pool be controlled?

Some pools have steps that descend progressively into the pool. Other pools have ladders that permit an equally controlled immersion. All pool users should be encouraged to use these, rather than making an uncontrolled entry or exit from the pool. Diving into shallow water depths should not be permitted. Additionally, if pool users are allowed to jump or dive in, then they need to be instructed to look out for other swimmers, and ensure they do not move into their pathway. To promote a controlled entry and exit from the pool the instructor should arrive early, and stay later, to supervise participants. In exceptional circumstances, where participants arrive early or stay later for a swim, a lifeguard should be present.

## How can electrical equipment be used safely on the poolside?

If electrical equipment is permitted for use on the poolside, it should be positioned a safe distance from the water edge. It should only be used if it is connected to a circuit breaker, that is, an industrial standard residual current device; equipment that is connected directly to the mains should not be used. If it is necessary to change tapes during the workout, then the instructor's hands should be dry. (Having music on a single tape is ideal.) Using batteries to operate stereo equipment is a much safer option, though batteries have a short life span and are therefore less economical. Some pools will not allow the use of electrical equipment on the poolside. It is essential to find out this information prior to arriving to take a session.

Electrical equipment used on the poolside will also be exposed to the humid environment, so it should be maintained and serviced more regularly to optimise its performance. All electrical equipment should be stored away from the poolside when not in operation. When it is moved to and from the poolside, it should be lifted safely by keeping the back straight, bending the knees and using the thigh muscles to lift it to an appropriate carrying height. Very heavy equipment should be lifted by more than one person or ideally moved to and from the poolside on wheels.

## What clothing should be worn?

Participants should wear a well-fitted swimsuit, and women with large busts are advised to wear a supportive bra under their costume. Baggy clothing or Bermuda shorts are not appropriate since they will hold water. Bikinis are generally not recommended, since movements need to be modified to keep them in place. Indeed, more time will be spent worrying about the whereabouts of the swimwear than focusing on the workout. Jewellery should not be worn during exercise, since it may cause an injury to another person or may be lost in the water.

Instructors should wear fitted clothing that does not restrict their movement but will allow all their body movements to be clearly visible to participants. A fitted T-shirt or vest top, leotard, well-fitted swimsuit or crop top worn with shorts or leggings would be appropriate.

## Summary

Consideration of the safety issues discussed throughout this chapter should be sufficient to assist the design and implementation of all water-based exercise programmes. However, each pool environment is unique. Different pools may suit different types of session. Therefore, rather than restrict an opportunity to provide activity, the session should be adapted to accommodate the pool differences. Sometimes it will be necessary to modify the exercises to accommodate individual requirements, sometimes it will be necessary to adapt the complete session. The key is being equipped with the knowledge to recognise how the programme can be adapted.

# SHORT ANSWER REVISION QUESTIONS

1. Name **SIX** potential differences between pool training environments.

2. State **THREE** considerations for working in a:
   (a) hydrotherapy pool
   (b) children's teaching pool
   (c) pool with a sloping floor
   (d) pool where the water overflows to poolside
   (e) pool with gullies/hand rails
   (f) pool where there is a space between the water rim and the edge of the pool

3. Describe appropriate clothing for:
   (a) the teacher in a pool environment
   (b) participants in a pool environment.

4. State **TWO** issues that relate to the use of electrical equipment on poolside.

5. Give an example of **TWO** rescue aids that may be found on poolside.

# DESIGNING A WATER-BASED
# EXERCISE PROGRAMME

PART THREE

# SELECTING A PROGRAMME FORMAT 5

## OBJECTIVES

By the end of this chapter the reader will be able to:

*   Name a range of different types of water-based sessions
*   Recognise appropriateness of different water-based sessions for different pool environments
*   Recognise a traditional approach to session structure to train all components of fitness
*   Recognise changes to session structure to meet different types of sessions
*   Identify changes to duration and intensity to accommodate different fitness levels.

## What type of programme is suitable for the general population?

For most exercisers a programme format that targets all the components of physical fitness will be most appropriate. This provides a more holistic approach to fitness and should therefore meet all requirements and satisfy most personal fitness goals. The traditional format outlined in table 5.1 will train all components effectively.

> ### NEED TO KNOW
>
>
>
> *   The type of programme selected needs to take into consideration the needs of the target group and also the specific safety considerations for different pool designs.

In addition, this type of programme can be adapted to suit the different pool environments. However, in a shallow teaching pool it is advisable to alter the approach to cardiovascular training. The traditional selection of cardiovascular exercises that are illustrated in Chapter 8 are best replaced with water walking activities. (Some general ideas for a water walking workout are provided in Chapter 13.) This minor adaptation will reduce the potential stress placed on the joints from jumping in shallower water and will maximise the safety and effectiveness of the workout.

However, more specific programmes that target just one or two of the components of fitness may be requested by some target groups and also by some employers. Pools offering a large variety of water-based sessions will always be looking for new approaches to expand their existing timetable.

| Table 5.1 | The traditional session structure | | |
|---|---|---|---|
| Programme | Fitness components trained in the main workout | Section structure | Appropriate pool environment |
| Traditional | Cardiovascular fitness<br><br>Muscular strength and muscular endurance | Warm-up component<br><br>Main workout (part 1) Cardiovascular training<br><br>Main workout (part 2) Muscular strength and endurance training<br><br>Cool-down component | Can be adapted to suit most pool environments<br><br>For teaching pools, replace any jumping and explosive movements with water walking exercises |

| Table 5.2 | Alternative approaches for water-based exercising | | |
|---|---|---|---|
| Programme | Fitness components trained in the main workout | Section structure | Appropriate pool environment |
| Water walking | Cardiovascular<br><br>Muscular endurance | Warm-up component<br><br>Main workout Water walking<br><br>Cool-down component | Teaching pool is ideal for this programme, although it can be adapted to suit most other pool environments |
| Circuit | Cardiovascular<br><br>Muscular strength<br><br>Muscular endurance<br><br>Flexibility (in cool-down) | Warm-up component<br><br>Main workout Circuit training<br><br>Cool-down component | Can be adapted to suit most pool environments<br><br>For teaching pools, limit the number of jumping and explosive movements |

| Table 5.2 | Alternative approaches for water-based exercising (cont.) | | |
|-----------|-------------------------|-----------------|------------------------|
| Programme | Fitness components trained in the main workout | Section structure | Appropriate pool environment |
| Step | Cardiovascular<br><br>Muscular endurance | Warm-up component<br><br>Main workout<br>Step training<br><br>Cool-down component | Must have a constant water depth or a pool with a mechanically altered floor<br><br>Not suitable in pools with sloping floors – the steps slide and further muscle imbalance can be created trying to maintain position of the step |
| Resistance | Muscular strength<br><br>Muscular endurance | Warm-up component<br><br>Main workout<br>Resistance training<br><br>Cool-down component | Can be adapted to suit most pool environments |
| Stretch and relax | Flexibility | Warm-up component<br><br>Main workout<br>Flexibility<br><br>Cool-down component | Hydrotherapy pool is ideal<br><br>Teaching pools with higher temperatures may be appropriate<br><br>Not appropriate in very cool pools |

Note: Careful consideration should be given to the structure, design and content of any of these training programmes to ensure they fully assist with the achievement of participants' personal fitness goals and are safe to perform in the pool environment.

# What other types of programme designs are available?

There is a variety of different types of session format, each designed to train one or more of the specific components of fitness. An outline of some of the different approaches to water-based training is given in table 5.2. However, the programmes identified should not be perceived as the definitive list. There are endless ways to vary each of the sessions and create a whole new programme. The key principle is that the programme implemented meets the personal fitness goals of the participants and is appropriate for the environment.

In addition, for all programmes the main workout should be preceded by a thorough and appropriate warm-up, and concluded by a thorough and appropriate cool-down.

To achieve the more holistic training of all the components of fitness, but using a different approach to the session, refer to the later chapters in this section of the guide. Each chapter explains how to structure the specific components and illustrates some appropriate exercises. Appropriate activities for the different approaches are also explained and illustrated. The exercises selected focus primarily on training apparently healthy individuals without any particular specialist requirement. However, most of the exercises can be adapted to suit more specialist groups. This can be achieved by varying their intensity. Guidelines are provided on how to progress each exercise and how to modify it to cater for different groups.

## NEED TO KNOW

The components of the session include:
- Warm-up
- Cardiovascular (CV) training
- Muscular, strength and endurance (MSE) training
- Cool down

There must always be a warm-up and cool down. Main components can change to suit different training needs and types of session.

# How should the water-based training programme be structured?

All water-based workouts must be structured safely and effectively to maximise the benefits of the activity and to reduce the risk of injury. It is therefore essential that appropriate time is allocated for warming up before the main workout commences, and for cooling down afterwards. It is also essential that the timing and intensity of the exercises selected for the main workout reflect the requirements of the target group.

| Table 5.3 An outline of the structure, duration and intensity of components for different target groups | Less fit and specialist groups | Intermediate fitness level and general groups | Advanced fitness level and sport-specific groups |
|---|---|---|---|
| Overall duration of the session | 35–45 minutes | 45 minutes | 45–60 minutes |
| Overall intensity of session components | Low | Moderate | High |
| Speed of movement | Relatively slow pace | Moderate pace | Relatively faster pace |
| Warm-up component (mobility, pulse-raising preparatory stretch and re-warming) | Comparatively low intensity and long duration 12–20 minutes | Moderate intensity and duration 10–15 minutes | Comparatively higher intensity and shorter duration 10 minutes |
| Main workout (aim to include some cardiovascular work and some muscular strength and endurance work) | Comparatively short duration and low intensity 10–15 minutes | Moderate duration and moderate intensity 20–30 minutes | Longer duration and higher intensity 30–45 minutes |
| Cool-down component (cooling down, post workout stretches, relaxation and remobilisation) | Comparatively long duration and low intensity 10–13 minutes | Moderate duration and intensity 5–10 minutes | Shorter duration and relatively higher intensity 5–10 minutes |

Note: These timings are only suggested as guidelines and are variable depending on the environment, the requirements of the individual/group, and the structural design of the main workout.

# SHORT ANSWER REVISION QUESTIONS

1. Name **THREE** different types of water-based sessions.

2. Name the **FOUR** main components of a traditional session structure.

3. Name the **TWO** components that are essential for any session.

4. Name the **TWO** components that can be altered or excluded for different training goals.

5. Give **THREE** examples of how the type of session may need to be adapted to suit different pool environments.

6. Describe some of the changes to duration and intensity that would need to be made to accommodate different fitness levels.

# DESIGNING A WARM-UP

6

## OBJECTIVES

By the end of this chapter the reader will be able to:

- State the purpose of a warm-up component
- Describe the effects of the different warm-up activities on the body – mobility, pulse-raising and stretching
- Identify appropriate activities and exercises to achieve the aims of each aspect of the warm-up in a water-based exercise session
- Recognise how the properties of water will affect the content and structure of the warm-up component
- Recognise methods of adapting the exercises within the warm-up to cater for different levels of ability and fitness.

## Why do we need to warm up before the main workout?

We need to warm up prior to activity to prepare all the bodily systems for the activity that will follow. Warming up will potentially enhance our performance and may reduce the risk of injury. A thorough warm-up should therefore help to maximise the safety and effectiveness of the activity. It is essential that appropriate time is set aside for warming up before the main workout commences. It is also vital that the correct exercises are selected. This chapter discusses what should happen to the body during this preparatory component of the session (the short-term physiological responses). It also outlines how to design a safe and effective warm-up and achieve the desired responses.

### NEED TO KNOW

The warm-up prepares the body for the exercises to follow.

## What type of exercises should the warm-up contain?

The warm-up needs to prepare the joints, muscles, heart, and the circulatory and neuromuscular systems for the main workout. It should therefore contain exercises that achieve the desired effects outlined in table 6.1.

| Table 6.1 | An outline of the desired effects of the warm-up on the body |
|---|---|

Warm-up exercises should be characterised by the following.

- They should promote the release of synovial fluid into the joint capsule and warm the tendons, muscles and ligaments which surround each joint. This will ensure the joints are adequately lubricated and cushioned, and will allow a fuller range of motion to be achieved at each joint. This can be achieved by **mobility exercises.**
- They should increase the heart rate, promote an increase of blood flow to the muscles and an increase in the delivery of oxygen. This will make the body warmer, the muscles more pliable and will allow them to work more comfortably throughout the main workout. This can be achieved by **pulse-raising exercises.**
- They should lengthen the muscles and move them through a larger range of motion. This will allow them to contract more effectively in the main workout and may lower the risk of injury if moving into extended positions in the main workout. This can be achieved by **stretching exercises.**
- They should activate the brain and neuromuscular pathways, focusing attention and concentration, rehearsing skills and movement patterns, rehearsing the muscle and joint actions in the way they are to be moved in the main workout, and raising the heart rate to a desired level. This can be achieved by **re-warming exercises.**

## What types of exercises are appropriate to mobilise the joints?

Moving each of the joint areas through their natural range of motion will achieve the desired effects listed in table 6.1. All of the joints to be used in the main workout should be targeted. Examples of the main actions of the joints and appropriate exercises for each joint area are outlined in table 6.2. The exercises selected should start with a small range of motion and progressively move to a larger range of motion. However, they should only ever be taken through a range of motion that is comfortable for the individual to achieve.

An example of progressively building the range of motion for the shoulder joint is to start with lifting and lowering the shoulders (elevation and depression), progress to rolling and rotating the shoulders, and finish by performing the larger movements such as taking the arms to the side of the body and back in (abduction and adduction), and circling the arm through the water, into the air and out of the water (circumduction). It should be noted that this is not intended to be the definitive guide on how to warm up this joint area, it is simply an example of how the range of motion can be progressed in one joint area.

## What joints should be mobilised?

The main selection of mobility exercises should be focused on preparing the specific joints that will be doing a majority of the work planned for the main session. On land, the primary focus should be on the lower body. This is because

| Table 6.2 | The actions possible at each joint area and appropriate exercises to achieve that action | |
| --- | --- | --- |
| **Joint area** | **Joint actions possible** | **Appropriate exercises** |
| Ankle | Plantar and dorsi flexion | • Heel and toe alternately pointing to the floor<br>• Walking/pedalling through the feet |
| Knee | Flexion and extension | • Bending and straightening the knees (Squats)<br>• Kicking the heel to the bottom |
| Hip | Flexion and extension<br><br>Abduction and adduction<br><br>Rotation | • Lifting the knees up towards the chest and down again<br>• Lunging the leg backwards and forwards (Spotty Dogs)<br>• Taking the leg out to the side and back in (Jumping Jacks)<br>• Circling one leg in towards the other leg and out again in a figure-of-eight motion |
| Spine | Lateral flexion and extension<br>Rotation<br>Flexion and extension | • Side bends<br>• Side twists<br>• Humping and hollowing the spine |
| Shoulder and shoulder girdle | Elevation and depression<br>Abduction and adduction<br><br>Rotation<br><br>Horizontal flexion and extension<br><br>Circumduction | • Lifting and lowering the shoulders<br>• Taking the arms out to the side of the body and back in<br>• Rotating the arm in a figure-of-eight motion towards and away from the body<br>• With the arms at shoulder level in a crucifix position, pulling forwards and backwards (Bear Hugs)<br>• Moving the arm in a complete circle (back stroke and front crawl) |
| Elbow | Flexion, extension and rotation | • Bending and straightening the elbow |

the joints in this area will be required to cushion the impact forces, and support most of the body weight during the main cardiovascular workout. But in water, buoyancy will cushion most of the impact forces, so the lower body is to some extent less of a priority in a water-based session. The resistance of the water usually requires the plentiful use of upper body propulsive movements to create movement and maintain balance. The upper body can also be used more effectively in the main workout when training for cardiovascular fitness. It may therefore be necessary to prioritise the mobilisation of the upper body in preparation for the water-based training session. However, this is dependent on how the main workout is structured.

Ideally, plan the warm-up after the plan for the main session activities. This will ensure that the body is appropriately prepared. It is neither safe nor effective to prepare purely the upper body, when in fact the lower body is doing a large proportion of the work in the main session. Ultimately, it is advisable to prepare all the joints, since it is unlikely that any joint area will receive no work at all in the main session.

through a larger range of motion more easily than they would if exercising on land. In addition, the movements for less fit and specialist groups may need to be performed at a slightly slower pace. More repetitions, or sets of repetitions, of the same exercises may be necessary for them to achieve the desired effect.

A fitter group may be able quite safely to start with a relatively large range of motion and should be able to progress this to a much fuller range of motion without any discomfort. They should also be able to work through to their full range of motion at a slightly faster pace, with fewer sets of repetitions for specific joint areas. In general they should be able to warm up their joints more quickly, due to their increased body awareness and more effective physiological responses to warm-up activities. However, it is essential even with fitter groups that the movements do not become too energetic and too large until the muscles are fully warm. There will be a greater risk of damaging the tissues that surround the joints (muscles, tendons and ligaments) if the range of motion is built up too quickly.

## How will mobility exercises alter for different groups?

The range of motion that we have at each joint can vary from one joint area to another. It can also vary from one person to another. The starting point of the first mobility activity will be dependent on the range of motion that the group and individuals possess.

A specialist group may need to start with a relatively small range of motion and may not be able to build to a very large range of motion. However, the buoyancy of the water will provide support to their movements, so it is possible that they will achieve movement

## How will pool temperature affect mobility exercises?

The temperature of the pool will also determine the starting point for the range of motion of mobility exercises. The muscles and other tissues that surround the joints are less pliable when they are cold. Therefore, attempting to move the joint areas through too large a range of motion too soon will increase the risk of injury to these tissues if they are not sufficiently warm. In a cooler pool it is advisable to commence with some gentle pulse-raising movements to get the body warm before moving the joints through too large a range of motion.

In a warmer pool the joints can be moved to a fuller range of motion slightly sooner. It will be safer to perform joint mobility exercises before any specific pulse-raising activities have occurred in a pool where the temperature is slightly warmer.

## What types of exercises are appropriate to raise the pulse?

Any rhythmical movement utilising the larger muscle groups will achieve the desired effects outlined in table 6.1. The movements selected need progressively to increase the heart rate and blood flow through the muscles. This will ensure that adequate oxygen is delivered to the muscles; this will be needed to fuel activities through the main session. It will also ensure that the muscles are sufficiently warm and safe to stretch. Moving to a larger range of motion and stretching before the muscles are sufficiently warm may provide an increased risk of muscle tearing.

There is a whole variety of movements that are appropriate to get the body warm and increase the heart rate in water. Jogging, Spotty Dogs, and Travelling Flick Kicks, to name but a few, are all very effective. These exercises are illustrated at the end of this chapter. On land, these activities would place a greater stress on the joints. They would therefore not be recommended as appropriate warm-up activities. They are best saved purely for the main workout when performed on land.

When they are performed in water, these exercises are much less stressful. This is because the buoyancy of the water reduces the impact forces, and subsequently reduces the stress placed on the joints while they are being performed. They can therefore be included quite safely within the warm-up component,

provided of course that they are performed in an appropriate water depth. However, it is worth noting that they may still need to be performed at a relatively lower intensity than they would need to be if they were performed in the main workout. This is to ensure they do not become too intense for the body to cope with at this early stage in the session. Performing the activities at a relatively slower pace, with a slightly smaller range of motion, and with comparatively less force being exerted by the exerciser, should lower the intensity and make each exercise more comfortable to perform. Ultimately, the level of intensity at which they can be performed will be dependent on the fitness level and individual requirements of the person performing them.

When exercising in water, a more energetic and fuller range of motion mobility exercises may also effectively elevate the heart rate. Figure Eights and Side Twists, which are also illustrated at the end of this chapter, are examples of mobility exercises that will also have pulse-raising effects. These exercises would be less effective at raising the heart rate on land because the muscles used would be working against very little resistance. Indeed, on land, only the lower body mobility exercises, that utilise the larger muscles and require the body weight to be transferred (such as hamstring curls), would be sufficiently effective to demand greater supplies of oxygen and warm the muscles.

In water, the use of the arms under the water can be very effective at raising the heart rate and getting the body warm. This is because they are working against the added resistance from the water and may recruit further help from the larger muscles of the chest and back to create movement. However, these movements will still need to be sufficiently large and utilise their full leverage and surface area to assist warming up and pulse-raising effectively. Small movements of the arm, such as bicep curls (bending and straightening the elbow) will have limited pulse-raising effects. This is because that exercise isolates the smaller muscles, and the comparatively small leverage of the lower arm demands less energy to move through the water.

It is equally essential that the pulse-raising movements selected make gradual demands on the body. They too should start at relatively low intensity and should progress to a moderate intensity. This can be achieved by starting out with a basic movement, such as Spotty Dog, but taking smaller strides with less rebounding out of the water. To build the intensity, the strides can become longer, the body can rebound slightly more energetically out of the water, and the arms can be used to push more strongly through the water. Once again the speed of the progression from one stage to another, and the level of intensity one needs to start at, is dependent on the fitness level of the group.

## How will pulse-raising exercises alter for different groups?

Less fit and specialist groups may need to start at a relatively low level of intensity. They may not need to progress to such a high level to get warm. Lower levels of intensity can be achieved by working with shorter levers, smaller surface areas, smaller ranges of motion and at a relatively slower pace.

Fitter groups could start at a relatively moderate level of intensity and finish at a much higher level. Higher levels of intensity can be achieved by working through a larger range of motion, using longer levers, with greater surface areas and moving at a slightly faster pace. However, it is worth noting for all fitness levels that if the warm-up or pulse-raising activities start at too high an intensity, then the muscles

may undergo an oxygen deficit (they will not be supplied with sufficient oxygen). If this occurs they will tire very quickly and will not be able to work effectively through the main session. This reiterates the necessity for the warm-up to be gradual and progressive for all fitness levels.

## What type of exercises will lengthen and stretch the muscles?

Exercises which allow the muscles to lengthen and relax are effective to achieve the desired responses outlined in table 6.1. Chapter 2 in Part One of this book details two types of stretching exercises that are appropriate for a water-based session. These are static stretches and moving stretches. Static stretches are those where the muscle is lengthened to a point where mild tension is experienced and then held still until the tension subsides. Moving stretches are those where the muscle is lengthened and moved slowly to a point where a mild tension is felt and then returned to its normal starting position. This process is generally repeated a few times so that each time the muscle should ease slightly further into an extended position.

An advantage of performing moving stretches in water is that they will assist with the maintenance of a comfortable temperature. Static stretches will tend to make the body cool down too quickly. If static stretches are preferred, then a larger proportion of pulse-raising movements performed between stretches will be necessary to keep the body warm. However, this will be dependent on the temperature of the pool. If working in a warmer pool on a warm day, the body will cool down less rapidly. Therefore, in these circumstances it is perfectly acceptable to perform all static stretches, and potentially a lower proportion of pulse-raising movements between stretches. But remember that if the muscles are allowed to cool down they will no longer stretch so effectively. Stretching cold muscles could also potentially cause them injury.

## Which muscles need to be stretched?

All the muscles to be used in the main workout should be lengthened prior to work. Prioritisation should obviously be given to those that will be working the hardest. On land, this would almost certainly be the muscles of the lower body, with the exception of a weight-training workout which specifically targets the upper body. However, in water the arms are used to perform propulsive movements to assist movement of the body through the water. Therefore, the upper body should receive equal focus in a water-based session. However, once again this will depend on the selection of exercises planned for the main workout. If the main workout contains a larger proportion of lower body-work, then obviously this area needs to be targeted slightly more. Ultimately, it is advisable to stretch all the muscles, since it is unlikely that a specific body area will not be used at all in the session. A range of appropriate stretches for each specific muscle group is illustrated at the end of Chapter 7.

## What type of stretch is most appropriate for each fitness level?

The type of stretch selected will be determined by the ability of the participants. Static stretches are potentially safer for those with lower skill levels and a smaller range of movement. This is because a safe range of motion is less likely to be exceeded when holding stretches in a static position, provided that the range of motion has not already been exceeded. If anything more than a mild tension is experienced, or if the muscle begins to shake, it is a sure sign that the stretch has been taken too far. It is advisable to reduce the range of motion slightly or move out of the stretch and try again, this time moving into the stretch position more carefully. However, static stretches will potentially cool the body down much quicker and this would need to be considered and accommodated by including more pulse-raising moves in between stretches.

Alternatively, moving stretches require greater body awareness to prevent a safe range of motion being exceeded. They are therefore more appropriate for those who are more experienced, have greater body awareness, and who have a larger range of movement. A key consideration is that the resistance of the water will prevent the range of movement being reached too quickly. This makes dynamic stretches more appropriate for most groups in a water-based session.

## What is the purpose of re-warming?

The body may have cooled down slightly after performing the preparatory stretches. It is therefore essential to re-warm the muscles before commencing the main workout. In addition, the re-warmer can be used to prepare the body more specifically for the main activity. It allows a rehearsal of specific movement patterns that will stimulate the neuromuscular pathways. This will help to improve the performance of all movements and enhance the effectiveness of the main workout.

## What type of exercise is appropriate for re-warming the body?

The movements to be used in the main workout are appropriate for re-warming. However, it is essential that the intensity of the movements starts at a relatively low pace and builds progressively to the level of intensity required for the main workout. This is to maximise use of the aerobic energy system and avoid unnecessary discomfort that may be experienced from using anaerobic energy systems as the primary fuel for movement. The latter is more likely to occur if the intensity starts too high, or builds too quickly. Ultimately, the intensity of the exercises will be dependent on the fitness level of the individuals, and the activities used within the main workout.

## How will the main workout affect the exercises selected for the re-warmer?

If the main workout is to comprise solely or predominantly of resistance training exercises (muscular strength and endurance), the exercises selected for the re-warmer should reflect this, but should be slightly less intense. For example, if flotation equipment is to be used in the main workout, it would be beneficial to perform the same exercises without the device within the re-warmer. If no flotation equipment is used in the main workout then performing the exercises with shorter levers, at an easier pace or with less force being exerted, will act as an effective rehearsal. However, it may also be necessary to incorporate some larger pulse-raising movements throughout this component in a resistance training session. This will ensure that a comfortable body temperature is maintained.

If the main workout is to comprise solely of cardiovascular or aerobic training exercises, then the movements in the re-warmer should resemble less energetic versions of those to be used in the main session. The exercises should start at a less energetic pace and progressively build to a higher level of intensity. For example, The Sploosh (*see* page 138) can start with no jump, progress to a small jump, then a higher jump, and can finish by jumping with a half or full turn. In practice, a sequence of movements should be selected and repeated three or four times, each time making the individual exercises a little harder, progressively raising the intensity.

## How will the re-warmer need to be adapted when dealing with different fitness levels?

A less fit or specialist group may need to start at a lower level of intensity, and the movements used throughout will need to be comparatively less intense. The exercisers will need to spend slightly longer building up the size of their movements to ensure the intensity is raised at a more gradual pace and their body is able to cope with the demands being made upon it.

Alternatively, a fitter group may start at a relatively higher intensity and work harder much sooner. They should not need to spend so long on this specific component. They can still work progressively to a higher level, but will be able to move at a higher intensity much sooner, because their cardiovascular system will more effectively deliver and utilise the oxygen they demand.

## How do the properties of water affect the content and structure of the warm-up?

- **Buoyancy** provides support for body weight. It will allow a higher proportion of jumping movements to be performed throughout the warm-up without placing the joints under unnecessary stress. It will also allow mobility exercises to be performed with relative ease and through a larger range of motion.
- **Resistance** will require all movements to be slower than on land, with fewer quick changes of direction. This resistance to movement prevents the end of the range of motion being reached too quickly. Therefore, moving stretches are much safer than on land. In addition, it will increase the pulse-raising effects of some upper body mobility exercises, primarily those that require the full leverage and surface area of the limbs to be pulled through the water.
- The **temperature** of the water and air will have a cooling effect on the body, making it harder to get warm and stay warm. Movements therefore need to be more active throughout the whole of the warm-up.
- **Hydrostatic pressure** will have a lowering effect on the heart rate but will also assist with the circulation of blood. This allows the intensity of the warm-up to be slightly higher than would be appropriate on land. It also allows for a steeper build-up of intensity. Therefore, the duration of the warm-up can be slightly shorter.

## What other factors affect the overall timing and intensity of the warm-up?

- Temperature of the water and air
- Fitness level
- Age of participants.

If the air and pool temperatures are cool, a longer duration should be allocated for warming up to ensure that the body is warm and that this is achieved gradually. In addition, many more large pulse-raising movements need to be incorporated throughout the warm-up to ensure the body remains sufficiently warm.

For lower levels of fitness, senior, and other more specialist groups, a longer warm-up with a more progressive graduation of intensity is needed. This is to ensure that the demands made upon the body are progressive and gradual and do not create an oxygen deficit. Specific adaptations to adjust the intensity of each individual stage of the warm-up, to accommodate different fitness levels and different environments, have been discussed throughout this chapter.

## How should the warm-up be structured for a water-based training session?

The warm-up should be structured in three stages:

1 Mobility and pulse-raising exercises (general warm-up)
2 Preparatory stretches and range of motion work
3 Re-warmer (specific warm-up).

## What is the appropriate posture?

- Spine lengthened and upright
- Shoulders relaxed and down from the ears
- Shoulder blades sliding down the ribcage towards buttocks

- Pelvis neutral – pubic and pelvic bones vertically aligned
- Abdominals engaged by visualising a zipping and hollowing feel from deep inside the tummy
- Head up, chin parallel and looking forward.

---

### SUMMARY OF THE GUIDELINES FOR PLANNING THE WARM-UP

Generally speaking, for all groups, the warm-up can be slightly more energetic and slightly shorter than it would need to be on land. This is primarily because the hydrostatic pressure assists circulation and will promote engagement of the aerobic energy system.

- Start with smaller mobility and pulse-raising exercises and gradually build up the range of motion and intensity of the movements. This can be achieved by progressively moving through a larger range of motion, increasing the length and surface areas of levers moved, and moving at a progressively faster pace.
- Activities traditionally described as high impact are LOWER impact in water; they can be included to assist with pulse-raising and may also contribute to mobility.
- Combine static mobility exercises with larger pulse-raising movements to maintain a comfortable temperature.
- Aim to use larger mobility exercises that require a longer lever to be dragged through the water to assist with the warming process e.g. Figure Eights.
- Ensure that the body is fully warm before stretching and moving to a larger range of motion.
- Combine static stretches with larger pulse-raising moves to keep warm.
- Incorporate, when possible, a larger percentage of full range of motion/dynamic stretches (moving stretches). Again, this will assist with the warming process.

# SHORT ANSWER REVISION QUESTIONS

1. State the purpose for the inclusion of:
   (a) mobility exercises in the warm-up
   (b) pulse-raising exercises in the warm-up
   (c) stretching exercises in the warm-up.

2. Give **TWO** examples of how the properties of water will affect the exercises selected in the water-based warm-up component.

3. Describe how the temperature of the pool may affect the warm-up structure and content.

4. Describe how the warm-up content and structure may need to be adapted for a low fitness level group.

5. State **TWO** considerations that may affect the choice of stretching method selected for the water-based warm-up component (static/dynamic).

6. List **TWO** factors that would affect the:
   (a) joints mobilised in the session
   (b) muscles stretched in the session.

7. What would be an appropriate time range for completing the warm-up in a water-based session?

8. List **FOUR** general guidelines for planning the warm-up in a water-based session.

# Exercises for the warm-up

## Exercise 6.1 • Figure Eights

| Exercise 6.1 | Figure Eights |
| --- | --- |

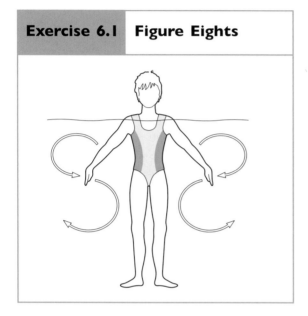

## Purpose

This exercise will mobilise the shoulder, elbow and wrist. If the movement is made progressively larger it will also assist with warming the muscles. It will provide dynamic range of motion lengthening for the latissiumus dorsi and oblique muscles. If performed with a greater intensity, it can be used in the main workout to improve cardiovascular fitness.

## Starting position and instructions

Select either a staggered or straddle foot position. Rotate the arm from the shoulder, in towards the middle of the body and out again in a figure-of-eight motion.

Repeat for the desired number of repetitions and then change arms.

## Coaching points

- Maintain an upright posture and engage the abdominal muscles.
- Slightly bend the knees.
- Slightly bend the elbows.
- As the body becomes warmer, start to bring in a humping and hollowing movement of the upper back.
- Keep movements of the lower back to a minimum.

## Progressions

- Start with the fingers open and progress to a cupped hand.
- Start slowly and increase the speed of the movement.
- Progressively exert greater force against the water in all directions.
- Progressively take the movement through a larger range of motion.
- Start by using each arm individually and progress to using both arms at the same time.

## Exercise 6.2 • Side Twists

| Exercise 6.2 | Side Twists |
| --- | --- |

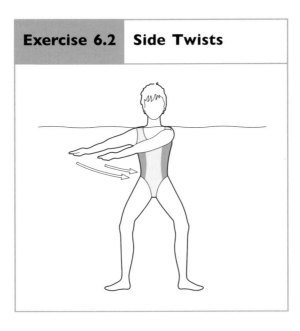

### Purpose

This exercise will mobilise the thoracic spine, shoulders and elbows. If the movement is made progressively larger it will also assist with warming the muscles. It will also provide dynamic range of motion lengthening for the latissiumus dorsi and oblique muscles. If performed with a greater intensity, it can be used in the main workout to improve cardio-vascular fitness.

### Starting position and instructions

Select either a staggered or straddle foot position. Use both arms to pull the water around to one side of the body and then back to the other side. Cup the hands to pull the water.

### Coaching points

- Keep the hips and knees facing forward. Do not let the knee joint roll inward.
- Keep the elbows slightly bent.
- Make sure the lower back does not twist.
- Keep the arms under the water.
- Maintain upright posture and engage the abdominal muscles.

### Progressions

- Start with fingers open or slicing the water with the side of the hand. Progress to a cupped hand.
- Start slowly, and progressively increase the speed of the movement.
- Progressively exert greater force against the water in all directions.
- Progressively take the movement through a larger range of motion, but maintain correct spinal alignment.

# Exercise 6.3 • Jog Heels to Bottom

| Exercise 6.3 | **Jog Heels to Bottom** |
|---|---|

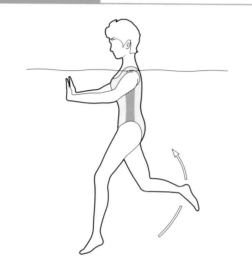

Note: This movement can be moved forwards through the water because the legs assist with pushing the water backwards. To travel back it is advisable to select a movement where the legs push the water forward, i.e. Flick Kicks.

## Purpose

This exercise will mobilise the knee joint and potentially, but to a lesser extent, the ankle. If the movement is made progressively larger it will also assist with warming the muscles. It will provide dynamic range of motion lengthening for the quadriceps muscles. It can be performed at a greater intensity and used in the main workout to improve cardiovascular fitness.

## Starting position and instructions

Select a straddle foot position where the feet are hip width apart and commence jogging and kicking alternate heels to the bottom.

## Coaching points

- Ensure the heels go down to the floor: this will maximise movement through the ankle and will prevent the calf muscles cramping.
- Kick the heels towards the buttocks, but only move to a range of motion that feels comfortable.
- Keep the hips facing forwards and ensure the heels do not kick to the outside of the buttock cheek. This may place unnecessary strain on the medial ligaments (the inner side of the knee joint).
- Keep the knee of the supporting leg unlocked.
- If the arms are used, ensure the elbows remain unlocked.
- Keep an upright posture and engage the abdominal muscles.

## Progressions

- Start with a smaller range of motion by kicking the heels only halfway towards the buttocks. Build to a full range of motion where the heels loosely touch the buttock cheeks.
- Increase the speed at which the movement is performed.
- Exert a greater force against the water with each movement of the lower leg.
- Use the arms to increase the number of muscle groups working.
- Move forward to increase the intensity.

## Exercise 6.4 • Spotty Dogs

| Exercise 6.4 | Spotty Dogs |
|---|---|

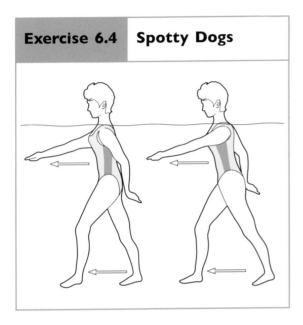

### Purpose

This exercise primarily assists with raising the pulse and warming the muscles. However, if the legs are moved through a progressively larger range of motion, it will also have a mobilising effect on the hip joint. It will provide dynamic range of motion lengthening for the calf muscles and muscles around the hip joint. If performed at a greater intensity it can be used in the main workout to improve cardiovascular fitness.

### Starting position and instructions

- Select a straddle foot position where the feet are hip width apart.
- Stride the legs alternately backwards and forwards.
- Use the arms in opposition to the legs.

### Coaching points

- Maintain upright posture and engage the abdominal muscles.
- Ensure the heels go down to the floor: this will maximise movement through the ankle and will prevent the calf muscles cramping.
- Care should be taken not to force the heel of the back leg to the floor, unless it feels comfortable. This could potentially cause a ballistic stretch of the calf muscle, depending on the flexibility of the individual, the speed of the movement, and the water depth.
- Stride the legs progressively to a larger range of motion, but only move through a range of motion that feels comfortable.
- Keep the hips facing forwards and avoid hollowing the lower back by tightening the abdominal muscles.
- Keep both knees unlocked. This will avoid placing any stress on the cruciate ligaments, which help to stabilise the knee joint.
- If the arms are used, keep the elbows unlocked.
- Keep arm movements under water to maximise effectiveness.
- Ensure movements of the shoulder joint are controlled.

### Progressions

- Start with small strides and increase to a larger range of motion by increasing stride length.
- Move at a progressively faster pace.
- Exert a greater force against the water with each movement of the lower leg.
- Use the arms in opposition to the legs: this will assist balance and increase intensity by working more muscles.

## Exercise 6.5 • Side Squats Pulling Water

| Exercise 6.5 | Side Squats |
|---|---|

Pull water

Travel

Note: It will be easier to stabilise during this exercise if a number of repetitions are performed in one direction and a static exercise (e.g. Spotty Dog) is performed before changing direction. This allows the eddy currents to subside and assists movement in the opposite direction.

### Purpose

This exercise primarily assists with raising the pulse and warming the muscles. If a wide stride is taken on the squat movement there may be some mobilisation benefits for the hip. In addition, the bending and straightening action of the knee will provide some mobilisation for this area. There may potentially be some mobilisation benefits for the shoulder and elbow joint from pulling the water away from the desired direction of travel (a propulsive action to assist movement). The elbows are required to bend and straighten throughout the movement and there is horizontal flexion and extension of the shoulder joint. If performed at a greater intensity, it can be used in the main workout to improve cardiovascular fitness.

### Starting position and instructions

Select a straddle foot position where the feet are hip width apart. Commence by stepping wider and squatting the legs apart, at the same time pulling the water away from the desired direction of travel. This will assist movement through the water.

### Coaching points

- Maintain upright posture and engage the abdominal muscles.
- Squat the legs progressively to a larger range of motion, but only continue while it feels comfortable and achievable.
- Keep the hips facing forwards and avoid hollowing the lower back by tightening the abdominal muscles.
- Avoid locking the knees as the leg straightens.
- Keep the elbows unlocked and the arms under water to maximise effectiveness. Ensure movements of the shoulder joint are controlled.

### Progressions

- Start with small strides and progressively increase the stride length to increase the range of motion.
- Start slowly and progressively move faster.
- Pull more forcefully against the water to create further travel and greater dragging.
- Perform fewer repetitions of the movement in the same direction, or perform a low number in one direction and then move back in the opposite direction. This will maximise work against the eddy resistance.

## Exercise 6.6 • Water Scoops

| Exercise 6.6 | Water Scoops |
|---|---|

Pull water

Travel ⟸

Note: It will be easier to stabilise during this exercise if a number of repetitions are performed in one direction and a static exercise (e.g. Jumping Jack) is performed before changing direction. This allows the eddy currents to subside and assists movement in the opposite direction.

### Purpose

This exercise primarily assists with raising the pulse and warming the muscles. If it is performed with a greater intensity, it can effectively be used to improve cardiovascular fitness.

### Starting position and instructions

Select a straddle foot position where the feet are hip width apart. Step diagonally forwards to the right corner of the pool. Pull the water away from the direction of travel, and drag the trailing leg through the water. Repeat, stepping diagonally forward to the left corner of the pool.

Perform these alternating diagonal scoops for the desired number of repetitions.

### Coaching points

- Take a large but comfortable stride.
- Keep the elbows slightly bent when pulling the water.
- Keep the hips facing forwards and avoid hollowing the lower back by tightening the abdominal muscles.
- Keep movements of the shoulder joint controlled.
- Keep an upright posture and engage the abdominal muscles.

### Progressions

- Start with a small stride and progressively increase stride length.
- Move at a progressively faster pace.
- Exert a greater force when pulling the water.
- Travel further through the water by increasing the number of repetitions.
- Perform fewer repetitions in the same direction and change direction of movement more quickly to increase eddy currents.

## Exercise 6.7 • Travelling Flick Kicks

| Exercise 6.7 | Travelling Flick Kicks |
|---|---|

Note: To perform this exercise and maintain a stationary position, pull the water backwards with the arms as the leg kicks forwards. Both movements need to be performed with equal intensity to prevent unwanted travelling.

## Purpose

This exercise primarily assists with raising the pulse and warming the muscles. It will also provide dynamic range of motion lengthening for the hamstring muscles if it is performed more slowly and through a greater range of motion. If it is performed with a greater intensity it can be used to improve cardiovascular fitness.

## Starting position and instructions

Select a straddle foot position where the feet are hip width apart. Hop on the right leg and at the same time kick the water forward with the left leg. Repeat this action, hopping on the left leg and kicking the water forward with the right leg. As each leg kicks forwards, a backwards travelling action should occur.

## Coaching points

- Keep the weight-bearing knee joint unlocked.
- Take care not to lock the knee as the leg kicks forwards.
- Keep an upright posture and engage the abdominal muscles.
- If the arms are used to push the water (and travel back) or pull the water (to keep stationary), keep the elbows slightly bent.
- Keep the arms under the water to maximise use of the water resistance.
- Keep the hips facing forwards and avoid hollowing the lower back by keeping the abdominal muscles pulled in tight.

## Progressions

- Start with a small hop and exert a little force when kicking and pushing the water.
- Progress to a larger hop and exert greater force to kick and push the water.
- Travel further backwards through the water by increasing the number of repetitions.
- Add a rebound out of the water and use the arms forcefully to push the water.

## Exercise 6.8 • Water Pushes

| Exercise 6.8 | Water Pushes |
|---|---|

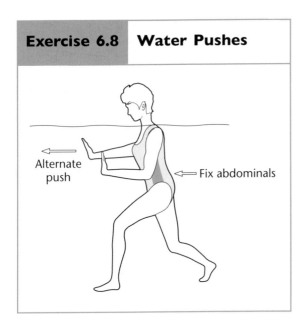

Alternate push

⟸ Fix abdominals

### Purpose

This exercise primarily assists with raising the pulse and warming the muscles. It may contribute to mobilising the shoulder joint if performed at a slower pace and through a slightly greater range of motion. If it is performed with a greater intensity, it can be used to improve cardiovascular fitness.

### Starting position and instructions

Select a staggered foot position where the feet are positioned hip width apart with one foot slightly in front of the other. Use the arms alternately to push the water forwards.

### Coaching points

- Keep the elbows and knees slightly bent throughout.
- Keep the arms under the water to maximise use of the water resistance.
- Keep the hips facing forwards and avoid hollowing the lower back by keeping the abdominal muscles pulled in.
- Keep an upright posture and engage the abdominal muscles.

### Progressions

- Start by exerting a little force when pushing through the water.
- Progress by exerting greater force to push the water.
- Move at a progressively faster pace to increase pulse-raising effects (slower to enhance joint mobility).
- Alternate speed of movements – quick, quick, slow, quick, quick, slow, or slow, slow, quick, quick, quick, quick.

# Exercise 6.9 • Jog High Knees

| Exercise 6.9 | Jog High Knees |
| --- | --- |

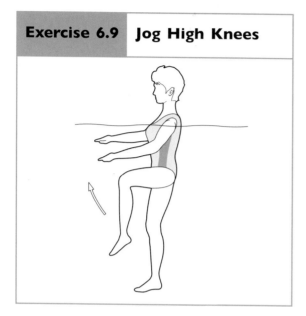

## Coaching points

- Maintain upright posture and engage the abdominal muscles.
- Ensure the heels go down to the floor. This will maximise movement through the ankle and will prevent the calf muscles from cramping.
- Raise the knees to the surface of the water, but only move to a range of motion that is comfortable.
- Keep the knee of the supporting leg unlocked.
- If the arms are used, ensure the elbows remain unlocked.

## Progressions

- Start with a smaller range of motion and build to a full range of motion where the knees raise towards the water surface.
- Extend the knees to lengthen the hamstrings.

## Purpose

This exercise will mobilise the hip joint and potentially, but to a lesser extent, the ankle. If the movement is made progressively larger, it will also assist with warming the muscles. It will provide dynamic range of motion lengthening for the gluteal muscles. If performed at a greater intensity, it can be used in the main workout to improve cardiovascular fitness.

## Starting position and instructions

Select a straddle foot position where the feet are hip width apart. Start jogging, raising the knees towards the surface of the water.

# SHORT ANSWER REVISION QUESTIONS

How could the following exercises be adapted or progressed for the specific needs/requirements listed below?

NB: Readers may need to refer to, and apply, information discussed in Chapter 1 to answer these questions.

1. Jog with high knees for overweight individuals with increased flotation/buoyancy.

2. Flick Kicks for individuals with less balance and lower skills for performing propulsive movements.

3. Figure Eights for individuals with less flexibility and range of motion.

4. Side Squats for individuals with larger mid section (e.g. pregnancy).

5. Side Bends and Spine Twists in a cooler pool environment.

# DESIGNING A COOL-DOWN

7

## OBJECTIVES

By the end of this chapter the reader will be able to:

- State the purpose of a cool-down component
- Describe the effects of the different cool-down activities on the body – pulse lowering and post-workout stretching
- Identify appropriate activities and exercises to achieve the aims of each aspect of the cool-down in a water-based exercise session
- Recognise how the properties of water will affect the content and structure of the cool-down component
- Recognise methods of adapting the exercises within the cool-down to cater for different levels of ability and fitness.

## Why is it necessary to cool down after a water-based workout?

We need to cool down after the main workout to return all the bodily systems back to their pre-exercise state. It is therefore essential that appropriate time is set aside for cooling down. At the end of the cool-down we should feel refreshed, rejuvenated and motivated to return, so the appropriate and correct exercises need to be selected. This chapter discusses what should happen to the body during this concluding component of the session (the short-term physiological responses), and also outlines how to design a safe and effective cool-down.

## What type of exercises should the cool-down contain?

The cool-down needs to include exercises that return the body to its pre-exercise state. It should contain exercises that will achieve the desired effects outlined in table 7.1 on page 108.

## What types of exercises are appropriate to lower the pulse and cool-down?

Exercises that progressively and gradually reduce the intensity of the activities used throughout the main workout will effectively lower the heart rate, breathing rate, and the body temperature. This can be achieved easily by starting the cool-down with larger movements, which continue the inten-

| Table 7.1 | An outline of the desired effects of the cool-down on the body |
|---|---|

Cool-down exercises should be characterised by the following:

- They should gradually return and lower the heart rate to a pre-exercise level. This reduces the stress on the heart muscle. It also promotes the return of venous blood to the heart and lowers the risk of blood pooling. This can be achieved by **pulse lowering/cooling down** exercises.
- They should lengthen the muscles back to their normal state. This will maintain the flexibility and range of motion of the muscles and joints. This can be achieved by **maintenance stretches.**
- They should increase the length of the muscles. This will increase the flexibility and range of motion of the joints and muscles. This can be achieved by **developmental stretches.**
- They should relax the body and mind. This will help to reduce stress and promote a feeling of serenity. This can be achieved by specific **relaxation** techniques.
- They should revitalise the body and mind. This will leave the body feeling rejuvenated and ready to return to normal activities. This can be achieved by gentle **re-mobilising** exercises.

sity of the main workout, and by gradually making each exercise less intense. Progressively reducing the speed of the exercises, performing them with shorter levers, and moving through a smaller range of motion, will lower the intensity of each movement. However, care should be taken not to reduce the intensity too quickly: this would give the heart little time to adapt and can be stressful and potentially dangerous. It is advisable to slow down gradually.

The physical properties of water assist the cooling down process. Firstly, the hydrostatic pressure will promote greater circulation of blood to the heart and the brain. The heart muscle is therefore provided some assistance with the return of venous blood during the cooling down phase. This reduces some of the stress placed on the heart and lowers the risk of fainting and dizziness that can occur if blood pools in the lower extremities. In addition, the temperature of the water will promote greater cooling of the body. As a consequence, the cool-down can be slightly shorter and the intensity can decline at a slightly faster rate than would

be safe to achieve on land. However, it is essential that the body temperature is not allowed to lower too much. So, while the intensity must be reduced, a sufficient number of moderate intensity movements need to be continued through the whole cool-down component. This will assist with the maintenance of a comfortable temperature and ensure that the body stays sufficiently warm to stretch safely.

## How will pulse-lowering and cooling down exercises alter for different groups?

Although less fit exercisers and specialist groups will be working at a relatively low intensity in the main workout, they will need to spend slightly longer cooling down because generally their body takes more time to recover from the demands of the workout. The cool-down for a less fit group will therefore need to start at a lower intensity, and more time should be spent on continuing to decrease it.

Fitter groups will be working at a higher intensity in the main workout but, despite this, they can still cool down at a more rapid pace because their body systems are more efficient. The intensity of the cool-down for a fitter group can therefore start at a much higher level and decrease more quickly. The intensity of warming movements maintained throughout the rest of the component will need to be relatively higher to keep them sufficiently warm.

## What types of exercises are appropriate to stretch the muscles?

Exercises that allow the muscles to relax and lengthen are appropriate here. This can be achieved by performing a combination of the same static or moving/dynamic stretches that are used for the preparatory (warm-up) stretch. Both types of stretch will fulfil the main requirement of the post-workout stretch, which is to lengthen the muscles after work and maintain their range of motion.

However, if static stretches are used, then it is advisable to perform warming movements between each stretch to keep the body sufficiently warm. Dynamic/moving stretches tend to be more effective at maintaining a comfortable body temperature, especially when working in cooler pool temperatures.

To improve flexibility, developmental stretches would need to be included in the cool-down. In a land-based session, developmental stretches are those where the muscle reaches a point where a mild tension is experienced and held still. When the tension eases, the muscles can then be lengthened further by moving to a greater range of motion. This process can be repeated a few times, moving even further into the stretch every time the tension eases. Once a comfortable, but extended, range of motion

is achieved the stretch should be held for as long as is comfortable. This will promote the achievement of a greater range of motion.

However, in a water-based session it is unlikely that the body will be able to maintain sufficient warmth to include developmental stretches, and the turbulence of the water may make it harder to maintain balance and hold positions comfortably. These stretches are therefore only recommended if comfortable positions are selected, and if the body is very warm. In most instances, it is advisable for the majority of post-workout stretches to be employed for the maintenance of flexibility and should be dynamic in nature.

## Which muscles need to be stretched after the main workout?

All muscles will need to be stretched and lengthened after work, so stretches should be included for all the muscles used in the main workout. The stretch positions illustrated at the end of this chapter can be used for pre-workout and post-workout stretching. However, it is generally advisable to make the post-workout stretch slightly less energetic and less active, by making the movements between stretches slower, more flowing and more relaxed. This will help to reduce the amount of physical tension in the body, and is more conducive to achieving the aims of the cool-down.

If the main workout is very intense, it can be effective to include extra stretches for the muscles that have worked hardest throughout. However, the level of activity and number of stretches included will also be dependent on the temperature of the water. If the water is cooler, then it is advisable to keep the cool-down more active and prioritise the number of stretches.

# What types of exercises are appropriate to relax the body and mind?

Exercises that do not require excessive muscular work, and activities which allow the mind to relax, are very effective in bringing about a relaxed state. There are various traditionally land-based relaxation techniques that can be used. These include the tense and release method, the extend and release method, and the visualisation method. Each method can be equally effective, so it is advisable to utilise a variety of the techniques.

## Tense and release

This can be achieved by tensing the muscles in a specific body area, holding for a short duration, and then releasing the tension, allowing the area to relax. For example, flexing the foot so that the toes point towards the knee will tense the muscle at the front of the shin (tibialis anterior) and relax the muscles of the calf (gastrocnemius and soleus). Working through each individual part of the body is preferable to tensing the whole body which can sometimes make you feel more tense.

## Extend and release

This can be achieved by extending the muscles in a specific body area, holding the position for a short time and then relaxing the position. For example, in a comfortable position, press the feet away from the head, hold the position, and then release the position.

## Visualisation

This can be achieved by mentally visualising a situation or place where you always feel relaxed. No specific scenario is recommended because each individual will react differently to different environments.

Ultimately, the suitability of specific relaxation techniques will depend on the temperature of the pool. In a warmer pool a longer duration can be spent on relaxation and can be very therapeutic. Relaxation activities are not appropriate in cooler pools. Three positions for relaxing in water are illustrated in Fig. 7.1.

# How will relaxation exercises alter for different groups?

It is possible that none of the positions illustrated will be relaxing for the participant who is nervous of the water. It is therefore advisable to provide equipment to assist their flotation, and to partner them with a confident swimmer to make them feel more comfortable. Some pools have very shallow water ledges, or a series of steps entering the pool at the shallow end: these are ideal for the less confident. They can sit or lie in this shallow water area and will relax more easily.

## Fig. 7.1a  Relaxing as a group

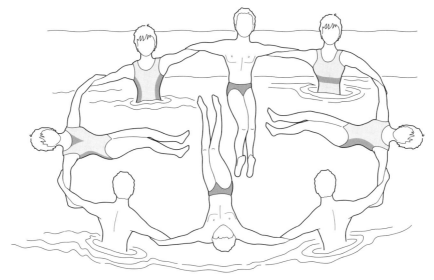

Note: There must be an even number of participants for this activity. The group should hold arms in a circle, and every second person should lie back and float and be supported by other group members. The members of the group who are standing can then walk slowly around in a circle.

## Fig. 7.1b  Relaxing with a partner

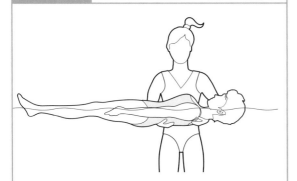

Note: One partner should support the weight of the other by positioning one hand between the shoulder blades and the other at the base of the lower spine. They can then move around the pool in any direction.

# What types of exercises are appropriate to revitalise the body?

At the end of the session participants should leave feeling refreshed, sufficiently warm, and motivated to return to another session. Therefore, lower intensity versions of the exercises illustrated at the end of Chapter 6, that are used for warming up, can be appropriate to re-mobilise the body. It can be quite effective to prepare a fun sequence to finish the session. This approach to revitalising usually works more effectively in water than it does on land. However, it is advisable to make any movements slightly less energetic at this stage of the session: the aim is not to prepare the body for a workout but to return to daily life.

| Fig. 7.1c | Relaxing alone |
| --- | --- |

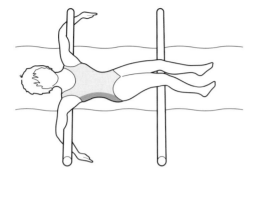

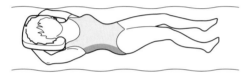 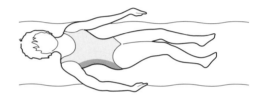

Note: Less buoyant body types may need to use a flotation device. Those who are very confident and comfortable in water may be quite happy to relax under the water for a short duration of time.

## How long should be spent on revitalising?

If a longer time is spent on specific relaxation exercises and static stretches, then a longer time will also be needed to revitalise the body. However, in most instances exercises that have a revitalising effect on the body need to be maintained throughout the whole component to maintain warmth. If this is the case then it will be unnecessary to set aside any further specific time for these particular activities.

## What other factors will affect the overall timing and intensity of the cool-down?

• The temperature of the pool and air
• The intensity of the main workout
• The age and ability of the participants.

The body will cool down much quicker when the pool and air temperature are cooler. Therefore, the cool-down will need to be kept shorter and comparatively more active in colder pools. This can be achieved by using fewer stationary movements (static stretches and relaxation exercises) and more active movements (moving stretches, mobility and gentle pulse-raising activities).

If the intensity of the main workout is relatively high, then a longer period of time will need to be spent lowering the intensity. If the preceding workout included a high proportion of cardiovascular activities, the intensity will need to start high and progressively decrease. If the preceding workout contained a higher proportion of muscular strength and endurance activities, then the cool-down will not need to start at such a high intensity, and less time will be needed to lower the intensity. Indeed, some less intense muscular strength and endurance activities may have a cooling effect on the body. Therefore, rather than cooling down, it may actually be necessary to re-warm the body prior to post-exercise stretching.

Less fit exercisers and specialist groups will need to spend slightly longer cooling down. However, the overall time can be comparatively shorter than would be needed for them to cool down after a land-based session. Fitter groups can also cool down much more quickly in water because the properties of water assist the whole cool-down process.

## SUMMARY OF HOW WATER AFFECTS THE CONTENT AND STRUCTURE OF THE COOL-DOWN

- Hydrostatic pressure will have a lowering effect on the heart rate and will also assist with the circulation of blood. This allows the intensity of the cool-down to be slightly higher than would be appropriate on land. It also allows for a steeper build down of intensity, so the duration of the cool-down can be slightly shorter.
- Buoyancy provides support for the body weight. It will allow a higher proportion of jumping movements to be performed throughout the cool-down without placing the joints under unnecessary stress. It will also provide support for stretching exercises and allow them to be performed with relative ease, so the muscles can be stretched more comfortably through a larger range of motion.
- Resistance will force all movements to be slower than on land, with fewer quick changes of direction. This resistance to movement prevents the end of the range of motion being reached too quickly. Therefore, moving stretches are much safer than on land. In addition, the range of motion stretches that require the full leverage and surface area of the limbs to be pulled through the water will have a warming effect on the body.
- The temperature of the water and air will cool the body down more rapidly. The timing and intensity of the whole component can therefore be lower. In addition, there will need to be more active movements throughout the component to keep warm. Any relaxation activities and developmental stretches should only occur in warmer pool temperatures.

## GUIDELINES FOR PLANNING THE COOL-DOWN

Generally speaking, for all groups the cool-down can be slightly shorter than it would need to be on land. However, the inclusion of specific warming movements to maintain a comfortable body temperature will be essential to prevent excessive cooling.

- Start with higher intensity exercises and gradually build down the range of motion and intensity of the movements. This can be achieved by progressively decreasing the length and surface areas of levers moved, continuing at a progressively slower pace and exerting less force against the water.
- Include a sufficient number of warming movements (moderate intensity pulse-raising activities) throughout the cool-down. This will help to maintain a comfortable temperature throughout the component.
- If static stretches are used, ensure that they are interspersed between sets of larger pulse-raising moves. This will ensure that the body is kept warm enough to stretch.
- Incorporate, when possible, a larger proportion of full range of motion stretches (moving stretches) to maintain flexibility. This will help to maintain a comfortable temperature throughout.
- Only include developmental stretches if the pool temperature is sufficiently warm, and then only if a stable position can be maintained.
- Only include specific relaxation exercises if the pool temperature is sufficiently warm.
- For re-mobilising, use larger range of motion mobility exercises that require a longer lever to be dragged through the water. This will assist with keeping warm.

## How should the cool-down be structured for a water-based session?

The cool-down component should be structured in four stages.

1 Cooling down/pulse-lowering exercises
2 Post-workout stretches: maintenance and developmental
3 Relaxation
4 Re-mobilisation.

The necessary adaptations to the content and intensity of each stage, for different fitness levels and different environments, have been discussed throughout this chapter.

# SHORT ANSWER REVISION QUESTIONS

NB: The reader may need to refer to the properties of water in Chapter 1 to answer these questions.

1. State the purpose for including pulse lowering as part of the cool-down from higher intensity cardiovascular (CV) training in a water-based session.

2. State **ONE** factor affecting the inclusion of static developmental stretches as part of the cool-down in a water-based session.

3. Explain **ONE** method of relaxation that can be used in the cool-down component in a water-based session.

4. Describe how the temperature of the pool and air temperature may affect the cool-down structure and content in a water-based session.

5. Describe how hydrostatic pressure may affect the activities included as part of the cool-down in a water-based session.

6. Describe how the cool-down content and structure for a water-based session may need to be adapted for a low fitness level group.

7. Give **ONE** reason why static stretches may be **LESS** beneficial for inclusion as part of the cool-down in a water-based session.

8. Give **ONE** reason why static stretches may be **MORE** beneficial for inclusion as part of the cool-down in a water-based session.

# Stretching exercises

**Note:** The stretch positions illustrated are appropriate for preparatory and post-workout stretching. The starting position and instructions are provided for both a dynamic/moving and static stretch.

## Exercise 7.1 • Back of Thigh Stretch

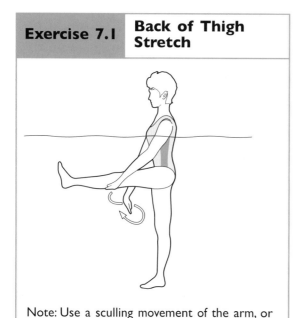

| Exercise 7.1 | **Back of Thigh Stretch** |
|---|---|

Note: Use a sculling movement of the arm, or hold on to the poolside to assist balance for static stretching.

### Purpose

This exercise lengthens and stretches the hamstring muscles at the back of the thigh, and also the buttock muscles (the gluteals).

### Starting position and instructions

**Static:** Balance on one leg. Allow the opposite leg to float towards the water surface. Use the hand to hold the leg and achieve a fuller range of motion; hold still.

**Dynamic:** Allow the leg to float to a point where a mild tension is felt, release out of the stretch and repeat. Or gently hop from one leg to the other, allowing each leg in turn to float through the water towards the surface to achieve a progressively larger range of motion.

### Coaching points

- Maintain upright posture and engage the abdominal muscles.
- Keep the weight-bearing knee joint unlocked.
- Only lift the leg to a point where a mild tension is felt at the back of the thigh.
- Keep the sculling arm under water with the elbow slightly bent.
- Keep the hips facing forwards and avoid hollowing the lower back.
- Aim to keep the knee joint of the leg stretched straight, but not locked.

### Progressions

- Start with a small range of motion by not lifting the leg very high.
- Progress to lifting the leg higher and closer to the water surface.
- Those with greater flexibility may be comfortable to lift the leg out of the water.
- Very flexible people may prefer to rest the leg on the pool wall or gully and bend the trunk of the body forward and over the leg to achieve a greater stretch.

## Exercise 7.2 • Front of Thigh Stretch

| Exercise 7.2 | Front of Thigh Stretch |
|---|---|

Note: Use a sculling movement of the arm, or hold on to the poolside to assist balance for static stretching.

### Purpose

This exercise lengthens and stretches the quadriceps muscles at the front of the thigh. If the hips are tilted forward, it will also stretch the hip flexor muscles (the iliopsoas).

### Starting position and instructions

**Static:** Balance on one leg. Raise the heel of the opposite leg towards the buttock cheek. Use the hand to hold the leg and achieve a fuller range of motion; hold still.

**Dynamic:** The legs can alternately float towards the buttocks, achieving a fuller range of motion each time. One leg can be stretched at a time by raising it towards the buttocks, lowering out of the stretch and repeating.

### Coaching points

- Maintain upright posture and engage the abdominal muscles.
- Keep the supporting knee joint unlocked.
- Only lift the leg to a point where a mild tension is felt at the front of the thigh: do not overflex (bend) the knee.
- Keep the sculling arm under water with the elbow slightly bent.
- Keep the hips facing forwards and avoid hollowing the lower back by keeping the abdominal muscles pulled in tight.
- Lift the heel towards the centre of the buttock cheeks. Avoid taking the heel to the outside of the buttocks as this may stress the ligaments on the inside of the knee.
- Tilt the hips slightly forwards.
- Keep both knees in line with each other.

### Progressions

- Start with a small range of motion by not lifting the leg very high.
- Keep the knee of the stretching leg slightly in front of the other knee to decrease the stretch.
- Progressively lift the heel closer towards the buttocks to achieve a greater range of motion.
- Tilt the hips forward to increase the stretch slightly.
- Take the knee of the stretching leg slightly back, so that it is positioned to the side but slightly behind the other knee to increase the stretch.

# Exercise 7.3 • Calf Stretch

| Exercise 7.3 | Calf Stretch |
|---|---|

Note: Keep the heel of the stretching leg on the pool floor and raise the toes upwards, placing the ball of the foot against the pool wall.

## Purpose

This exercise lengthens and stretches the gastrocnemius and soleus muscles at the back of the lower leg.

## Starting position and instructions

**Static:** Hold on to the pool wall with both hands. Keep one foot on the pool floor to balance.

Keep the heel of the other leg on the pool floor and lift the ball of the foot off the floor and rest it against the pool wall. Use the arms to pull the body closer to the wall and achieve a greater stretch of the calf muscles. The position illustrated is not so appropriate for performing a moving stretch. Moving into and out of the position will have little warming effect on the muscle. Therefore, a static stretch in this position is more appropriate and quicker.

**Dynamic:** An alternative moving stretch is to perform very slow and controlled Spotty Dogs (illustrated in Chapter 6) that progressively build to a larger range of motion and encourage the heel of the rear leg to extend gently and ease towards the pool floor. Care should be taken not to force the heel down, and the exercise should be performed in sufficiently deep water to maximise the support of the water.

## Coaching points

- Keep the knee joint of both legs unlocked.
- Only raise the ball of the foot to a point where a mild tension is felt in the calf.
- Keep the hips facing forwards and avoid hollowing the lower back by tucking the buttock muscles under.
- Keep an upright posture and engage the abdominal muscles.

## Progressions

- For a smaller range of motion, place the foot at a smaller distance up against the wall and do not ease the body so close to the wall.
- Lift the toes higher to achieve a greater range of motion.
- Use the arms to pull the body closer to the wall to achieve a greater range of motion.

## Exercise 7.4 • Inner Thigh Stretch

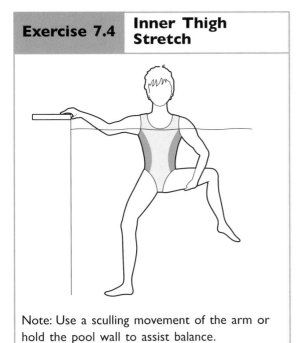

| Exercise 7.4 | Inner Thigh Stretch |
|---|---|

Note: Use a sculling movement of the arm or hold the pool wall to assist balance.

### Purpose

This exercise lengthens and stretches the adductor muscles at the inside of the thigh.

### Starting position and instructions

**Static:** Balance on one leg. Allow the other leg to lift and float out to the side of the body.

Use the hand to turn the knee out further. Hold still.

**Dynamic:** To perform as a moving stretch, move gently into and out of the position a few times, but only to a point where a mild tension is experienced. Alternatively, perform a very slow, low intensity version of the Farmer Giles exercise illustrated in Chapter 8, to move the adductor muscles through their range of motion.

### Coaching points

- Keep the knee joint of the supporting leg unlocked.
- Only raise the leg to a point where a mild tension is felt on the inner thigh and groin.
- Keep the hips facing forwards and avoid hollowing the lower back by tucking the buttock muscles under.
- Keep the sculling arm under the water and the elbow soft.
- Keep an upright posture and engage the abdominal muscles.

### Progressions

- Start with a smaller range of motion by lifting the leg to a lower height and by not turning the leg out so far.
- Progress by lifting the knee higher and rotating the hip out further to achieve a greater range of motion.
- Performing the stretch by facing the poolside, resting one foot in the gully of the pool or on the pool wall, and easing the body closer to the wall, will increase the stretch for those who are very flexible.

## Exercise 7.5 • Side Stretch

| Exercise 7.5 | Side Stretch |
|---|---|

Note: It is not recommended that the illustrated position be performed as a moving stretch, because the arm and muscles being stretched may be positioned out of the water, and affected by gravity. In addition, moving in this position will have little effect on the maintenance of a comfortable temperature. It is safer to perform this statically. The only exception would be for those with sufficient body awareness to maintain the control necessary to ensure the range of motion was not exceeded and a ballistic stretch did not occur.

### Purpose

This exercise lengthens and stretches the muscles at the side of the trunk and side of the back (the obliques and latissimus dorsi).

### Starting position and instructions

**Static:** Stand side-on to the poolside with the feet about one-and-a-half hip widths apart. Hold on to the poolside with the hand closest to the wall. Lift the other arm up and bend over to the side slightly.

### Coaching points

• Keep the knee joint of both legs slightly bent.
• Emphasise lifting the body upwards, and stretch to a point where a mild tension is felt at the side of the trunk.
• Keep the hips facing forwards and avoid hollowing the lower back by tucking the buttock muscles under.
• When bending to the side, move the body in a straight line and do not lean forwards or backwards.
• Lift the ribcage upwards and create a gap between the pelvis and the ribs before bending to the side.
• Keep an upright posture and engage the abdominal muscles.

### Progressions

• Start by only reaching the arm up and not bending over to the side.
• Progress by reaching the arm higher and bending over slightly further to achieve a greater range of motion.
• Those with greater flexibility can reach and touch the poolside with the arm that is stretching over, but the correct alignment of the spine must be maintained.

## Exercise 7.6 • Back of Upper Arm Stretch

| Exercise 7.6 | **Back of Upper Arm Stretch** |
|---|---|

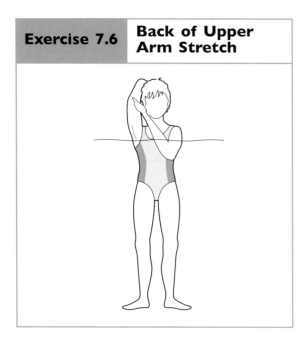

### Purpose

This exercise lengthens and stretches the triceps muscles at the back of the upper arm.

### Starting position and instructions

**Static:** Adopt either a staggered or straddled foot position. Place one hand either on the shoulder or in the centre of the back, and use the other arm to ease the arm upwards and stretch further; hold still.

**Dynamic:** The position illustrated is less effective at warming the muscles when performed as a moving stretch. For a more effective moving stretch, perform slow bending and straightening movements of the elbow, with the arms at shoulder height, the arms under the water, and the palms of the hands moving towards and away from the chest. Allow the buoyancy of the water to assist the movement.

### Coaching points

- Keep the knee joint of both legs slightly bent.
- Keep the hips facing forwards and avoid hollowing the lower back by tucking the buttock muscles under.
- Stretch only to a point where a mild tension is felt.
- Keep an upright posture and engage the abdominal muscles.

### Progressions

- Start with the hand on the shoulder. Ease the arm back slightly by using the other arm.
- Progress by placing the palm of the hand in the centre of the back and using the other arm to ease further into the position.
- Progress further by taking the other arm behind the back into a half-Nelson position and attempt to reach the fingers of the stretching arm. This will stretch the deltoid muscles at the front of the shoulder of the other arm.

## Exercise 7.7 • Chest and Middle Back Stretch

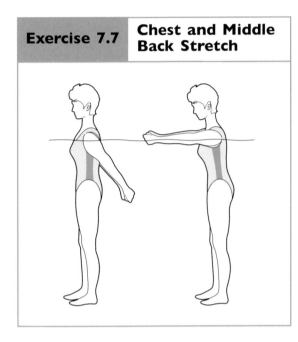

| Exercise 7.7 | **Chest and Middle Back Stretch** |

### Purpose

Position (a) lengthens and stretches the muscles of the chest (the pectorals). Position (b) stretches the muscles in the middle of the back (the trapezius).

### Starting position and instructions

Adopt a staggered or a straddled foot position.
**Static**: To perform as a static stretch, hold at both front and rear ends of the range of motion.
**Dynamic**: To perform as a moving stretch, allow the arms to float out to the side of the body and to the surface of the pool. Move the arms slowly forwards through the water, rounding the shoulders slightly and bending the neck forwards to feel a mild tension in the middle of the back, and back of the neck. Reverse the movement, taking the arms back-wards through the water and as far back as possible, lifting the chest up and forwards to stretch the muscles of the chest.

### Coaching points

• Keep the knees and elbows slightly bent.
• Keep the movement slow and controlled, and allow the arms to glide through the water.
• Keep the arms under the water.
• Keep the hips facing forwards and avoid hollowing the lower back by tucking the buttock muscles under.
• Engage abdominals to maintain balance.

### Progressions

• Start with a small range of motion.
• Move the arms progressively through a greater range of motion.
• Wrapping the arms around the body at the front with the hands touching the back (hug yourself) will increase the stretch for the trapezius.
• Taking the arms further back, allowing the hands to touch the buttocks and squeezing the shoulder blades together, will increase the stretch for the pectorals.

## SHORT ANSWER REVISION QUESTIONS

1. Describe both a dynamic stretch and a static stretch for the:
   (a) hamstrings
   (b) adductors
   (c) calves
   (d) quadriceps
   (e) pectorals.

# DESIGNING A CARDIOVASCULAR TRAINING PROGRAMME

## OBJECTIVES

By the end of this chapter the reader will be able to:

- Identify different approaches to training cardiovascular fitness in water
- Recognise a safe and effective session structure to improve cardiovascular fitness
- Recognise the effects of the properties of water on session content and structure
- Describe different approaches to cardiovascular training – continuous, fartlek and interval training
- Recognise a range of safe and effective exercises for inclusion in the cardiovascular component of a water-based session
- Explain the requirements for building up and building down intensity
- Recognise methods of adapting the exercises within the cardiovascular session to cater for different levels of ability and fitness
- Describe different methods of monitoring exercise intensity.

## How should the complete session be structured?

There are a variety of different approaches to cardiovascular training in water. Water walking, water-based step training, circuit training and deep-water training are a few of the approaches available. The structure of these specific sessions should follow the same format regardless of the approach adopted. A thorough warm-up and stretch should precede the main workout, and a warm-down should conclude the session. An appropriate structure is outlined in table 8.1.

However, the exercises selected will need to be adapted to suit each different approach. To improve the fitness of the heart, lungs and circulatory system, the activities selected for the main workout need to be performed at a higher level of intensity and should create a feeling of mild breathlessness – *see* ACSM guidelines for target heart rate listed in Chapter 2, table 2.1, page 31.

This chapter discusses how to structure a specific component to achieve safe and effective cardiovascular training in a water-based exercise session. Additionally, it illustrates a variety of exercises that can be performed when exercising in chest depth water. A range of exercises for water-based step training is illustrated in Chapter 9.

| Table 8.1 | The structure of a session to train cardiovascular fitness |
|---|---|

Specifically to train to improve cardiovascular fitness, the session should comprise the following components:

**Warm-up**
- Mobility and pulse-raising activities.
- Preparatory stretches.

**Main workout (1): cardiovascular training (essential)**
- Re-warmer to raise the intensity.
- Maintenance of intensity at appropriate level.
- Warm-down to lower intensity and promote venous return.

**Main workout (2): muscular strength and endurance training (optional)**
- Specific toning exercises for muscles not targeted in main session.

**Cool-down**
- Post-workout stretches.
- Relaxation activities (optional).
- Re-mobilise.

# What activities are appropriate to re-warm the body and increase the intensity for cardiovascular training?

The re-warmer component should commence with less intense versions of the activities to be performed in the main component. The intensity of each exercise will then need to be progressively built up to the desired level. This can be achieved by starting with relatively smaller movements, and gradually increasing the size of the movement. Moving the centre of buoyancy/gravity progressively in either an upwards, downwards or travelling direction, are effective methods of increasing the intensity to improve cardiovascular fitness. Increasing the length of the moving levers (the arms and legs), the speed of movement, and the force exerted against the water, is also very effective.

# What factors will affect the rate at which the intensity can be increased?

The rate at which the intensity can be progressed will be dependent primarily on the fitness of the participants. Less fit exercisers and specialist groups will generally need slightly longer than would be required by a fitter group. However, for all groups, the intensity can build up at a slightly faster pace than would be appropriate on land. This is due to the effects of the hydrostatic pressure on the body. This pressure promotes the circulation of blood and has a lowering effect on the heart rate. It therefore tends to promote more effective usage of the aerobic energy system.

The progressive graduation of this component will also be dependent on the intensity maintained throughout the preparatory stretch. If the body is kept fairly active, and the intensity is maintained at a reasonable level throughout that component, then it is unlikely that so much time will need to be spent re-warming. The intensity can therefore be raised to a higher level at a slightly faster pace.

# What activities are appropriate to maintain the intensity?

Exercises that require the use of the larger muscle groups, and maintain a constant intensity and a mild state of breathlessness, are appropriate here. Oxygen consumption is generally higher during travelling moves, due to the shifting of the centre of buoyancy and the whole of the body's resistance through the water. The increased resistance to movements will place a greater demand on the muscular systems when creating movement through the water. This, in turn, will make demands on the cardiovascular system to deliver more oxygen. Most of the activities illustrated at the end of this chapter can be travelled through the water, so they are very effective for maintaining intensity. In addition, Flick Kicks and Travelling Side Squats (*see* pages 101–3), can also be effective if they are performed at a higher intensity.

Movements that require the body to be lifted out of the water, such as Tuck Jumps and Leap Frogs (illustrated at the end of this chapter) will be effective. However, they are also very demanding and generally cannot be performed at a high intensity for a long duration. It is therefore effective to combine these more explosive movements with travelling movements through the water, and movements that use the arms intensely under the water, such as Water Pushes (*see* Ex 6.8, page 104).

# How will fitness levels affect the intensity maintained?

The intensity, and the duration for which it is maintained, will be very much dependent on the level of fitness of the participant. Less fit exercisers and specialist groups will need to work at a lower intensity and for an overall shorter duration than would a fitter group. They should perform their higher intensity exercises at less frequent intervals throughout the component. This will allow them time to recover and feel comfortable throughout the workout.

A fitter group should have a more effective cardiovascular system. They should therefore be able to work at a higher intensity for a longer duration, so any higher intensity activities can be performed at more frequent intervals, and a comparatively longer time can be spent performing each activity. The duration of the whole component can also be slightly longer.

It is worth reiterating at this point that an activity that is easy for a fitter group may well be very intense for a less fit and specialist group. Therefore, careful consideration should be made when selecting the intensity for lower fitness levels. It is advisable to exclude the higher intensity exercises, such as those that lift the body explosively out of the water, when dealing with these groups. These activities demand a greater skill level and are also very demanding. However, a range of progressions are detailed for all the exercises illustrated at the end of this chapter. It may therefore be appropriate to offer a modified version of the more intense activities. As a guideline, the intensity of most movements can be reduced by performing the exercise using shorter levers, moving at a slower pace, exerting less energy, and travelling slightly less.

# What training approaches can be used to structure the main component?

## Continuous training

Continuous training involves maintaining the heart rate at the appropriate level of intensity (target heart rate zone), below the anaerobic threshold for at least 20 minutes with the intention of developing aerobic capacity. Maintaining a constant intensity is much easier when using cardiovascular machines, where a set intensity level and speed can be established. Exercise intensity within a water-based session can be maintained at a steady state but this is very much dependent on the choreography and type of exercise used! The introduction of new moves and visual previewing of any new choreography will, to some extent, alter the intensity and should be considered when selecting the desired training approach.

## Fartlek training

Fartlek training involves playing with the speed. The resistance of the water, to some extent, limits the amount of speed variations that can be performed comfortably in a water-based session. However, speed can still be varied with regard to the resistance of the water by adapting the surface area of different body levers (arms and legs) to enable different movement speeds to be achieved more easily.

In addition, varying the choreography or type of movements selected will, by nature, create a fartlek approach to some extent.
For example:
- 8 Travelling Side Squats – slow pace
- 8 Sploosh and Turn – faster pace and more explosive
- 16 Runs forward – moderate pace
- 8 Jumping Jacks – moderate pace
- 16 Runs back – moderate pace
- 16 Sprint Runs on spot – faster pace.

## Interval training

Interval training involves the performance of specifically timed, shorter, higher intensity work periods in between blocks of specifically timed, lower intensity rest and recovery periods. The aim is to engage all the energy systems, however, the predominant system will be determined by the duration, intensity and type of exercise included for the work and rest intervals respectively.

Interval training can be achieved by using a circuit approach to exercise in water (*see* Chapter 12 which describes different circuits using specifically timed work and rest intervals).

Work interval exercises, designed specifically to challenge the anaerobic energy systems, will need a shorter work time allocated and a longer and less active rest phase to enable replenishment of energy sources (ATP-CP). An appropriately calculated rest interval slows down the build-up of lactic acid, enabling the overall workload to be maintained. Energy systems and the effects of water on energy (e.g. hydrostatic pressure) are explored in Chapter 2 on page 32 and also within Chapter 1, page 20.

### Example interval using circuit approach:

Jogging around pool in a circle =

| Active rest interval | : | for 60–90 seconds (approx.) |
|---|---|---|

| Higher intensity work stations | : | Performed for 30–40 seconds (approx.) |
|---|---|---|

1. Sploosh
2. Sprints
3. Tuck Jumps
4. Leap Frogs
5. Deep-Water Tread Water
6. Deep-Water Press-ups out of water

## How will I know how hard the activity is?

There are various ways of monitoring the intensity of an activity. Heart rate monitoring is one

| Table 8.2 | Maximal heart rate and training zone for a 30-year-old |
| --- | --- |

220 – 30 (age) = 190 beats per minute (maximum heart rate)
10 per cent of this maximum = 19 bpm (approx.)

To calculate the training zone, multiply 19 (10 per cent of the maximal heart rate) by 5.5 (55 per cent) and 9.0 (90 per cent)

55 per cent of this maximum = 104 bpm (approx.)
(Calculation: 10 per cent of maximal heart rate x 5.5)

90 per cent of this maximum = 171 bpm (approx.)
(Calculation: 10 per cent of maximal heart rate x 9.0)

Therefore, the training zone for a 30-year-old would be between 104 and 171 bpm. That is, they should work between this range in the main workout to improve their cardiovascular fitness.

method. Maintaining the heart or pulse rate somewhere between 55 per cent and 90 per cent of its maximum beats per minute is suggested as an appropriate training range by the ACSM. The ACSM guidelines are explained in Chapter 2, table 2.1. An individual's maximum heart rate can be estimated by subtracting their age from 220. For example, a 30-year-old's maximal heart rate would be 190 beats per minute (*see* table 8.2).

## What factors will affect heart rate monitoring in water?

Accurate heart rate monitoring is never easy and is complicated further when exercising in water. Firstly, the turbulence of the water makes it difficult to obtain an accurate reading when taking the pulse manually. Secondly, the properties of water will naturally have a lowering effect on the heart rate. Therefore, the reading obtained may not be accurate. Two alternative methods for monitoring the

intensity that are more appropriate for a water-based session are the talk test and the perceived rate of exertion.

### NEED TO KNOW

- Hydrostatic pressure improves circulation, and heart rates in water tend to be lower.
- Turbulence will affect ability to monitor heart rate.
- Other methods of monitoring intensity may be easier in water.

## Talk test

Working to a level where one can breathe comfortably, rhythmically and hold a conversation while exercising is suggested to indicate an appropriate intensity. A guideline for using the talk test is provided in table 8.3.

| Table 8.3 | Using the talk test to monitor intensity | |
|---|---|---|
| Intensity level | Talk test response while performing an exercise | Action |
| Too high | If one or only a few words can be spoken | Lower the intensity immediately |
| Too low | If a number of sentences can be spoken too comfortably | Increase the intensity |
| Appropriate | If a mild breathlessness is apparent at the end of speaking a couple of sentences | Maintain this level of intensity |

## Perceived rate of exertion

Alternatively, Borg (1998) researched and developed two scales from which individuals could rate the intensity of exertion (*see* table 8.4). These scales provide a range of intensity levels from 0–10 and 6–20. An easy to remember verbal expression is used to suggest how the intensity of an activity is perceived by the performer. When the activity is perceived to be 'strong' (a rating of 4–7 on the CR10 scale and 13–16 on the RPE scale) Borg suggested these ranges should correspond to an appropriate intensity for improving cardiovascular fitness.

Monitoring intensity during water-based exercising is another area where more specific research and further guidelines are needed. The accuracy of the aforementioned approaches is questionable. They should therefore only be used to provide a guideline as to how hard a person is working. It is perhaps advisable to use a combination of the methods and be vigilant for signs of over-exertion such as heavy breathing and excessive pallor or flushing of the skin.

## When might it be necessary to stop exercising?

Exercise should be stopped, and it would be advisable to consult a doctor, if:
• normal co-ordination is lost while exercising
• dizziness occurs during exercise
• breathing difficulties are experienced
• tightness in the chest is experienced
• any other pain is experienced.

## What types of activities are appropriate to cool down and lower the intensity?

Exercises that progressively slow down the heart rate and breathing rate are appropriate. Commencing with the activities used to maintain the intensity, and progressively making the movements less intense, will achieve the desired effect. This can be reached by reducing the number of jumping and travelling movements, moving at a slower pace, exerting less energy, and utilising shorter levers.

| Table 8.4 | The Borg Rating of Perceived Exertion (RPE) 6–20 scale and the Borg Category Ratio – 10 (CR10) scales | | | | |

| RPE Scale | | CR10 Scale | | | |
| --- | --- | --- | --- | --- | --- |
| 6 | No exertion at all | 0 | Nothing at all | No P | |
| 7 | Extremely light | 0.3 | | | |
| 8 | | 0.5 | Extremely weak | Just noticeable | |
| 9 | Very light | 1 | Very weak | Light | |
| 10 | | 1.5 | | | |
| 11 | | 2 | Weak | | |
| 12 | | 2.5 | | | |
| 13 | Somewhat hard | 3 | Moderate | Strong | |
| 14 | | 4 | | | |
| 15 | Hard (heavy) | 5 | Strong | | |
| 16 | | 6 | | | |
| 17 | | 7 | Very strong | | |
| 18 | | 8 | | | |
| 19 | Extremely hard | 9 | Extremely strong | Max P | |
| 20 | Maximal exertion | 10 | | | |
| | | 11 | Absolute maximum | Highest possible | |

Borg, G. (1998) in ACSM (2006)

# What factors will affect the intensity and duration of the cool-down?

Hydrostatic pressure improves the circulation of blood around the body. The exercising heart rate will probably be lower, and the return of venous blood to the heart will be assisted. There will be less risk of blood pooling in the lower extremities when exercise is stopped. Therefore, a comparatively shorter duration will need to be spent on lowering the heart rate and promoting the venous return. Additionally, the intensity can be reduced at a slightly faster rate than would be appropriate on land. However, this is also determined by the fitness level of the participant.

A less fit group will need to spend slightly longer cooling down, even though they would not have been working at such a high intensity in the main workout. This is to allow their bodies sufficient time to recover. Alternatively, a fitter group should generally recover at a quicker rate and so they should be able to cool down more quickly.

## How can the programme be adapted for work in deep water?

When exercising in deep water, the effects of the properties of water will be greater. All the exercises illustrated at the end of this chapter can be adapted for use in a deep-water session. The principles listed below should be applied to ensure the programme is achievable.

• Movements will need to be much slower.

• More time will be needed for directional changes.
• Movements should be repeated for longer (fewer movement changes).
• Most exercises will need to be performed in a suspended state. Rebounding movements will be very intense and will require great effort to lift the body out of the water. They should only be performed by those fit enough and skilled enough to perform them.
• Buoyancy belts will be needed to assist flotation, although fitter groups can progress by performing some exercises without buoyancy equipment.
• Stronger propulsive movements will be needed to create travel. Travelling movements will also be more intense.

**Note:** Deep-water training may not be suitable for specialist groups, in particular pregnant women or non-swimmers.

---

### SUMMARY OF THE EFFECTS OF WATER ON THE CARDIOVASCULAR COMPONENT

**Hydrostatic pressure** promotes the circulation of blood around the body and has a lowering effect on the heart rate. It also assists with the return of venous blood (blood in the veins) to the heart. Therefore, the re-warmer and cool-down can ascend and descend respectively at a slightly faster pace.

**Buoyancy** reduces the impact forces on the body and supports the body weight. Therefore, it is safer to include a higher proportion of jumping and leaping movements, provided the water depth is appropriate.

**Resistance** increases the intensity of movements.
• Using the arms under the water will effectively challenge cardiovascular fitness.
• All movements need to be performed at a slower pace.
• More time will be needed to change direction.

---

# SHORT ANSWER REVISION QUESTIONS

NB: readers may also need to refer to the properties of water discussed in Chapter 1 to answer these questions.

1. Name **TWO** types of water-based programmes that specifically focus on training cardiovascular fitness.

2. What is the target heart rate training range suggested by the ACSM?

3. Give **ONE** reason why it is essential to build the intensity gradually for cardiovascular training in a water-based session.

4. Give **ONE** reason why it is essential to lower the intensity gradually after cardiovascular training in a water-based session.

5. State **TWO** ways of adapting the content and structure of the cardiovascular component in a water-based session to accommodate a lower fitness group.

6. Describe the **INTERVAL** method of training.

7. Describe the effects of hydrostatic pressure on the cardiovascular training component.

8. Describe the effects of buoyancy on the cardiovascular training component.

9. Describe how the resistance of water will affect movement in a water-based session.

10. State **THREE** ways of monitoring intensity in a water-based session.

11. State the advantages and disadvantages of different approaches to monitoring intensity in a water-based session.

# Exercises for the cardiovascular component

Most of the exercises illustrated can be used to increase, maintain, or decrease intensity. They can also be modified to suit different fitness levels. Refer to the suggested progressions to ensure the intensity selected is appropriate.

For all exercises maintain an upright posture and engage abdominal muscles (*see* posture guidelines described in Chapter 6 page 95).

## Exercise 8.1 • Rocking Horse

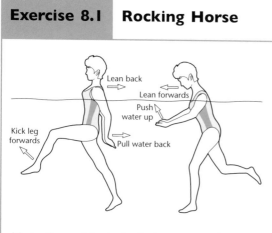

| Exercise 8.1 | Rocking Horse |
|---|---|

Lean back
Lean forwards
Push water up
Kick leg forwards
Pull water back

Note: If travel is desired, the water will need to be pulled away from the desired direction of travel. To travel forwards, the water should be forcefully pulled backwards, and vice-versa.

### Purpose

This exercise will elevate and maintain the heart rate. If performed at a lower intensity, it can be used in the warm-up session as a pulse-raising exercise.

### Starting position and instructions

Select a staggered foot position where one foot is placed in front of the other. Rock forwards taking the body weight on to the front leg, and curl the heel of the trailing leg towards the buttocks. Reverse the action by rocking backwards on to the rear leg, extending the knee, and kicking the water with the other leg. As the body rocks forwards, pull the water back with the arms; as the body rocks backwards, push the water forwards with the arms. These opposing propulsive movements will prevent unwanted travelling.

### Coaching points

- Ensure the heels go down to the floor to prevent the calf muscles cramping.
- Keep the weight-bearing knee joint unlocked.
- Keep the hips facing forwards and abdominals tight.
- Keep the elbows unlocked and the arms under water.

### Progressions

- Start with a smaller leverage, keeping the knees bent to move through the water.
- Progress by extending and straightening the legs to increase the leverage.
- Initially take small leaps; progress to taking larger strides.
- Exert more force with both the arms and legs to push and kick the water.
- Take the movement forwards in the water.

## Exercise 8.2 • Farmer Giles

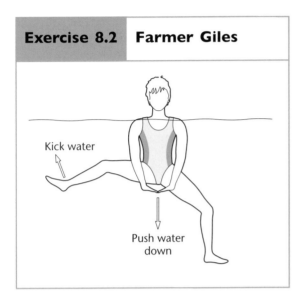

| Exercise 8.2 | Farmer Giles |
|---|---|

### Purpose

This exercise will elevate and maintain the heart rate. If performed at a lower intensity, it can be used in the warm-up as a pulse-raising exercise.

### Starting position and instructions

Adopt a wide leg straddled stance. Rock the body weight over on to one leg and lift the knee of the other leg. Then rock to the other side, taking the weight on to the other leg and lifting the other knee. The arms should be used in a pumping action, pushing the water down each time the weight is transferred.

### Coaching points

- Keep the weight-bearing knee joint unlocked.
- Take care not to lock the knee as the leg extends to the side.
- Keep the elbows slightly bent.
- Keep the arms under the water to maximise use of the water resistance.
- Keep the hips facing forwards.

### Progressions

- Start with just the knee lifting to the water surface, and progress to kicking the toes out of the water.
- Start by taking smaller jumps to each side and progressively make these larger.
- Exert more force with the arms and legs to push and kick the water.
- Progress further by extending the arms and pushing the water in the opposite direction of the kicking leg: this will alter the appearance of the movement.

## Exercise 8.3 • Leap Frogs

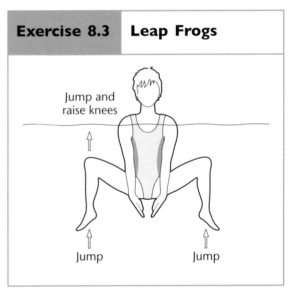

| Exercise 8.3 | Leap Frogs |
|---|---|

### Purpose

This is a high intensity exercise that should be used in the main workout. It should be combined with other exercises of a moderate to high intensity to improve cardiovascular fitness.

## Starting position and instructions

Adopt a wide straddled foot position. Bend the knees slightly and push through the thigh muscles to create an upward motion through the water. The knees should move towards the armpits. Use the arms to push the water down. This will assist the height of the movement.

## Coaching points

- Keep the knee joint unlocked.
- Ensure the heels go down when landing.
- Keep the elbows slightly bent throughout the movement.
- Keep the arms under the water to maximise use of the water resistance.
- Keep the hips facing forwards.

## Progressions

- Start with a small leap by pushing less forcefully through the thigh muscles.
- Progress to a larger leap by exerting a greater force to leap through the water.
- Use the arms more forcefully to increase the height of the jump.
- Move the exercise through the water.

# Exercise 8.4 • Tuck Jumps

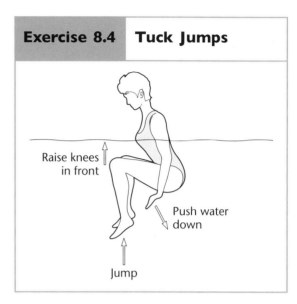

| Exercise 8.4 | Tuck Jumps |
|---|---|

## Purpose

This is a variation of the Leap Frog. It is another high intensity exercise that should be used specifically in the main workout. It should be combined with other exercises of a moderate intensity to improve cardiovascular fitness.

## Starting position and instructions

Adopt a narrow straddled foot position. Bend the knees and push through the thigh muscles to create an upward motion through the water. The knees should move to the front of the chest. The arms can be used to push down through the water and assist the height of the movement achieved.

## Coaching points

- Keep the knee joint unlocked.
- Ensure the heels go down when landing.
- Keep the elbows slightly bent throughout the movement.

- Keep the arms under the water to maximise use of the water resistance.
- Keep the hips facing forwards.

## Progressions

- Start with a small tuck by pushing less forcefully through the thigh muscles.
- Progress to a larger tuck by exerting a greater force to leap through the water.
- Use the arms more forcefully to increase the height of the jump and increase the overall intensity of the movement.
- Travel the movement.

## Exercise 8.5 • Pike Jumps

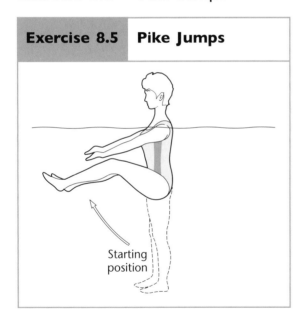

| Exercise 8.5 | Pike Jumps |
|---|---|

Starting position

## Purpose

This is a variation of the Tuck Jump. It is a very high intensity exercise that should be used specifically in the main workout. It should be combined with other exercises of a more moderate intensity to improve cardiovascular fitness.

## Starting position and instructions

Adopt a narrow straddled foot position. Bend the knees and push through the thigh muscles to create an upward motion through the water. The knees should move to the front of the chest and the legs can be extended. The arms can be used to push down through the water to assist the height of the movement achieved, and can reach towards the feet.

## Coaching points

- Keep the knee joint unlocked.
- Ensure the heels go down when landing.
- Keep the elbows slightly bent throughout the movement.
- Keep the arms under the water to maximise use of the water resistance.
- Keep the hips facing forwards.

## Progressions

- Start with a smaller jump by pushing less forcefully through the thigh muscles.
- Progress to a larger jump by exerting a greater force through the water.
- Use the arms more forcefully to increase the height of the jump and increase the overall intensity of the movement.
- Extend the knees straighter to increase the intensity of the movement.

## Exercise 8.6 • Gazelles

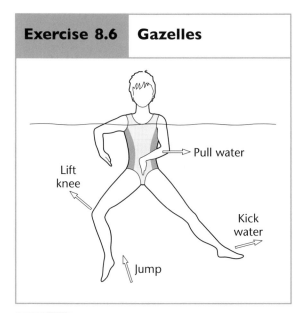

| Exercise 8.6 | Gazelles |
| --- | --- |

### Purpose

This exercise will assist with elevating and maintaining the intensity. It is a moderate intensity exercise that, if combined with other exercises of a higher intensity, will improve cardiovascular fitness.

### Starting position and instructions

Adopt a narrow straddled foot position. Bend the knees and push through the thigh muscles to create an upward and sideways travelling motion through the water. The legs should move in a leaping motion through the water. The arms can be used to pull through the water and achieve movement in the desired sideways direction.

### Coaching points

- Keep the knee joint unlocked.
- Ensure the heels go down when landing.
- Use the arms to pull through the water.
- Keep the elbows slightly bent throughout the movement.

- Keep the hips facing forwards.
- Push forcefully through the thighs.

### Progressions

- Start with a small leap by pushing less forcefully through the thigh muscles.
- Progress to a larger leap by exerting a greater force through the thighs.
- Use the arms more forcefully to increase the height and travel of the movement.
- Adapt to a side squat to reduce impact further.

## Exercise 8.7 • Jumping Jacks

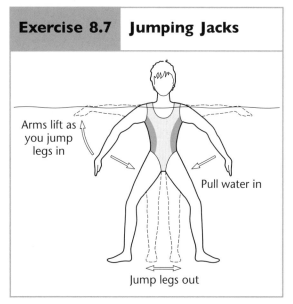

| Exercise 8.7 | Jumping Jacks |
| --- | --- |

### Purpose

This is a moderate intensity exercise that can be used to elevate and maintain the heart rate. If performed at a lower intensity it can be used within the warm-up as a pulse-raising exercise. If performed at a slower pace and through a fuller range of motion, it may contribute to mobilising the shoulders and hips within a warm-up.

## Starting position and instructions

Adopt a narrow straddled foot position. Bend the knees and push through the thigh muscles to jump the legs to a wider straddled position. The arms can be used to pull through the water and achieve greater height and movement out of the water.

## Coaching points

- Keep the knee joint unlocked.
- Ensure the heels go down when landing.
- Ensure the knee travels in line with the toe and over the ankle.
- Keep the elbows slightly bent throughout the movement and the hands cupped.
- Keep the hips facing forwards and the abdominals tight.

## Progressions

- Start with little rebound out of the water.
- Progress by exerting a greater force through the thighs and arms to jump further out of the water.
- Travel the movement forwards by using breast stroke arms to pull the water forwards.
- Travel the movement backward by pushing the water forwards with both arms.

# Exercise 8.8 • Sploosh

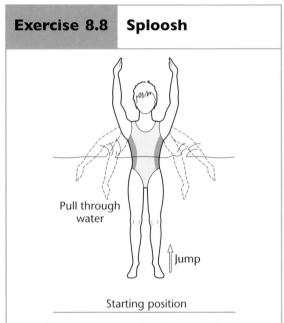

| Exercise 8.8 | Sploosh |
|---|---|

Pull through water

Jump

Starting position

Note: For participants who do not wish to sploosh the water over their head, allow them to lift the arms in front of the body and, if necessary, keep the arms lower, even under the water. In addition, care should be taken to control the arm movements. Uncontrolled arm movements crossing the surface may lead to a shoulder injury.

## Purpose

This exercise will elevate and maintain the heart rate. It can be either a moderate or high intensity exercise, depending on the height of the jump and whether turning movements are included.

## Starting position and instructions

Adopt a narrow straddled foot position. Bend the knees and push through the thigh muscles to jump out of the water. Use the arms to pull through the water and achieve greater height and movement out of the water. As the body lifts out of the water, the arms should be high and splooshing the water into the air.

## Coaching points

- Keep the knee joint unlocked.
- Ensure the heels go down when landing.
- Keep the elbows slightly bent throughout the movement and the hands cupped to pull through the water.
- Keep the hips facing forwards.

## Progressions

- Start with a small jump and little rebound out of the water.
- Progress to a larger jump out of the water by exerting a greater force through the thighs and using the arms strongly.
- Add a quarter, half or full turn when leaping out of the water to further increase the intensity of the movement.

# Exercise 8.9 • Treading Water

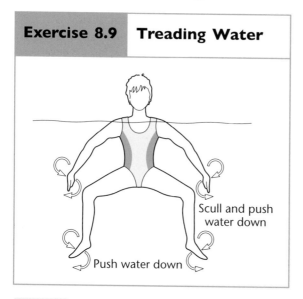

| Exercise 8.9 | Treading Water |
|---|---|

Scull and push water down

Push water down

## Purpose

This exercise will maintain the heart rate. It is performed in a suspended state and therefore requires greater effort to assist flotation. It is a higher intensity exercise.

## Starting position and instructions

Suspend the body so that the legs are not in contact with the pool floor. Use the hands to push the water down to assist flotation. Use the legs to push the water down to further assist maintenance of a suspended state.

## Coaching points

- Keep the knee joint unlocked.
- Keep the elbows slightly bent and the arms low under the water, level with the hip.
- Keep the hips facing forwards.

## Progressions

- Start with a small pedalling action of the legs and progress to a larger pedalling action.
- Exert a greater force through the thigh and the arms.
- Use flotation equipment to assist suspension then more effort can be used to perform the leg movements through a fuller range of motion.
- Perform in deep water. Aim to progress by trying to lift and push the body out of the water.

## Exercise 8.10 • Jogging

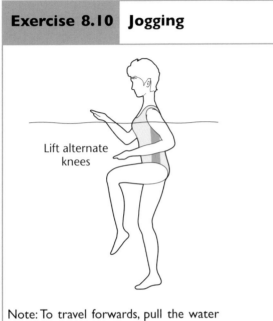

| Exercise 8.10 | Jogging |
|---|---|

Note: To travel forwards, pull the water backwards. To travel backwards, push or pull the water forwards.

### Purpose

This exercise primarily assists with raising and maintaining the heart rate.

### Starting position

Adopt a narrow straddled foot position. Commence lifting the legs in the water.

### Coaching points

- Keep the knee joint unlocked.
- Keep the elbows slightly bent if the arms are used throughout the movement.
- Keep the hips facing forwards.
- Ensure the heels go down.

### Progressions

- Start with a lighter jog.
- Progress by lifting the knees higher and in front of the body.
- Rebound the body out of the water in taking each stride.
- Jog at a slightly faster pace.
- Push more forcefully through the thighs.
- Use the arms to push down through the water and this will increase the number of muscles being worked.
- Add travel.

## Exercise 8.11 • Pendulums

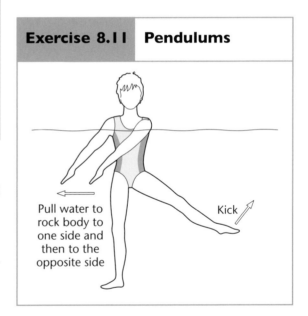

| Exercise 8.11 | Pendulums |
|---|---|

### Purpose

This exercise primarily assists with raising and maintaining the heart rate.

### Starting position

Adopt a narrow straddled foot position. Hop on one leg, swinging the other leg to the side of the body, and taking both arms across the front of the body, away from the swinging leg. Repeat by hopping on the other leg and moving the arms in the opposite direction.

## Coaching points

- Keep the knee joint unlocked.
- Keep the elbows slightly bent and the hands cupped.
- Keep the hips facing forwards.
- Ensure the heels go down.

## Progressions

- Start with a small hop and low leg swing.
- Progress by hopping slightly higher and swinging the leg out further.
- Rebound the body out of the water in taking each stride.
- Move at a slightly faster pace.
- Push the water more forcefully with the arms.
- Use the arms to push down through the water and this will increase the number of muscles being worked.
- Add travel.

# Exercise 8.12 • Ballet Jumps

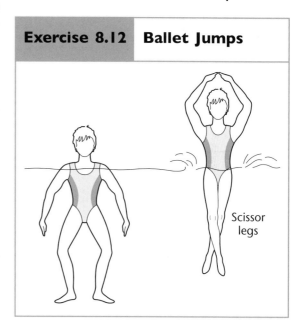

| Exercise 8.12 | Ballet Jumps |

Scissor legs

## Purpose

This exercise can be combined with other exercises of a more moderate intensity to improve cardiovascular fitness.

## Starting position and instructions

Adopt a narrow straddled foot position. Bend the knees and push through the thigh muscles to create an upward motion through the water. Criss-cross the legs on the upward phase of the movement. The arms can be used to help lift the body out of the water. They can also be positioned in a ballerina style.

## Coaching points

- Keep the knee joint unlocked.
- Ensure the heels go down when landing.
- Keep the abdominals pulled in.
- Keep the hips facing forwards.

## Progressions

- Start with a smaller jump by pushing less forcefully through the thigh muscles.
- Progress to a larger jump by exerting a greater force through the thighs.
- Use the arms more forcefully to increase the height of the jump and increase the overall intensity of the movement.
- Try and increase the number of leg criss-crosses while in the air.

## Exercise 8.13 • Shoot Ball

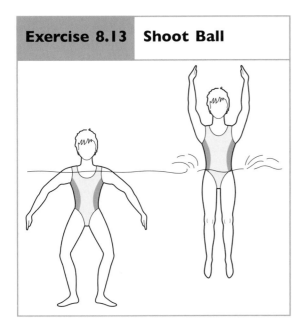

**Exercise 8.13** | **Shoot Ball**

## Purpose

This exercise can be combined with other exercises of a more moderate intensity to improve cardiovascular fitness.

## Starting position and instructions

Adopt a narrow straddled foot position. Bend the knees and push through the thigh muscles to create an upward motion and jump out of the water. The arms lift out of the water as if shooting a basketball into a net.

## Coaching points

- Keep the knee joint unlocked.
- Ensure the heels go down when landing.
- Keep the elbows slightly bent throughout the movement.
- Keep the abdominals pulled in throughout.
- Keep the hips facing forwards.

## Progressions

- Start with a smaller jump by pushing less forcefully through the thigh muscles.
- Progress to a larger jump by exerting a greater force through the thighs.

## SHORT ANSWER REVISION QUESTIONS

How could the following exercises be adapted or progressed for the specific needs/requirements listed below?

1. Sploosh for individuals with low motor skills.

2. Tuck Jumps for individuals with higher fitness levels.

3. Ballet Jumps for individuals advised to avoid hip adduction.

4. Pike Jumps for individuals who are overweight and/or have low hamstring flexibility.

5. Gazelle Leaps for individuals who have lower levels of balance in water.

# DESIGNING A WATER-BASED STEP TRAINING PROGRAMME

## OBJECTIVES

By the end of this chapter the reader will be able to:

- Recognise step training in water as a variation for training cardiovascular fitness and endurance
- Recognise some advantages and disadvantages of using step training in water
- Identify some ways water will affect step training
- Describe some basic methods of using step training in water (choreography).

## Why step in water?

Step training in water provides an alternative and effective method of training to improve cardiovascular fitness. It can provide variety for those who regularly exercise in water and may attract interest from other exercisers. Ideally, one should be reasonably skilled at manipulating the water and so move efficiently around the step. However, most of the movements can be adapted so that they are appropriate for, and achievable by, most participants.

## How should a water-based step programme be structured?

The water-based step programme should follow the same structural design as any other programme that targets cardiovascular fitness (*see* Chapter 8, table 8.1, page 125).

Ideally, the step should be utilised in all components of the session to avoid any unnecessary disruptions to the flow of the class. However, it is perfectly safe to use the steps only for the main workout. An advantage of including their use in the warm-up is to orientate participants to their whereabouts. In addition, movement patterns that will be used in the main workout can be introduced at a lower intensity, which allows any specific water skill advice to be provided. It is also safe to remove the steps from the pool prior to any muscular strength and endurance or cooling down activities, but this needs to be managed effectively so that participants do not cool off too much.

## How will water affect step training?

Buoyancy will reduce most of the impact forces. Therefore, a larger proportion of jumping movements on, off, over, and around the step are much safer. When stepping on land, these activities need to be limited because they are very high impact and place greater stress on the joints.

The resistance water provides to all movements

will require much effort to overcome. Therefore, a greater proportion of propulsive arm actions may be needed to assist movement onto and around the step. The resistance will also add intensity to both arm and leg movements, improving their muscular endurance. The use of water mitts is recommended in a step-training programme, to improve the effectiveness of propulsive movements, and to optimise muscular benefits.

## What is an appropriate water depth for step training?

Ideally, the water should be at chest depth when standing on the pool floor, and just above waist level when standing on the step. This water depth will maximise the use of the arms in the programme. If shallower water is used, it is advisable to include a muscular strength and endurance component specifically targeting the upper body, which would have received comparatively less work.

## What activities are appropriate for water-based step training?

There are five different ways of performing movements in a step-training programme. Specific exercises are illustrated and explained at the end of this chapter.

### Floor-based movements – not using the step

Floor-based movements can be used as a transitional move between different step patterns. Most of the cardiovascular exercises illustrated at the end of Chapter 8, and the warm-up exercises illustrated at the end of Chapter 6, can be used. Some of these exercises can also be adapted and performed in one or more of the other ways listed below.

### Basic – step-based

Adapting the basic form of each movement so that a basic step pattern is performed to move on and off the step. For example: Jogging becomes Run Up and Run Down.

### Rebound – step-based

Performing each movement on and off the step with the body lifting and rebounding out of the water. For example: Jumping Jacks become Straddle Jacks.

### Neutral – step-based

The body maintains a neutral position with just the head out of the water, and all movements lightly tap the step. The body stays low and under the water as each move is executed. For example: Spotty Dogs become Ski Strides.

### Suspended/buoyant – over the step

The body is suspended in a buoyant state over the top of the step, and the movement pattern is executed without the feet contacting the floor or the step. For example: Treading Water becomes Water Tread.

## SHORT ANSWER REVISION QUESTIONS

1. State **TWO** advantages of using step training in water.

2. State **TWO** disadvantages of using step training in water.

3. Describe **THREE** ways water will affect step training.

4. Describe **TWO** types of movements that can be used to create water step choreography.

## Water-based step training exercises

### Exercise 9.1 • Straddle Jacks (rebounding)

#### Purpose

This rebounding exercise will elevate and maintain the heart rate.

#### Starting position and instructions

Stand on top of the step. Jump the legs out to each side, straddling the step on landing. Let the arms move out to the side and raise them to the surface of the water. Push through the thighs to bring the legs together and return the feet on to the step. Use the arms to push down through the water to assist the movement on top of the step.

#### Coaching points

- Ensure feet are placed in the centre of the step.
- Ensure the heels go down.
- Keep the knee in line with the toe and over the ankle.
- Keep the elbows slightly bent and the hands cupped.
- Keep the hips facing forwards.

| Exercise 9.1 | Straddle Jacks (rebounding) |
|---|---|

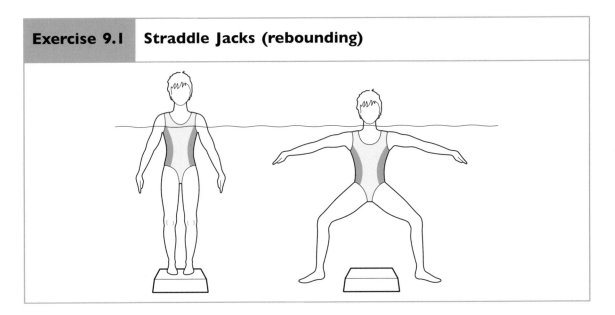

## Progressions

- Allow buoyancy to assist the move and rebound minimally.
- Rebound more forcefully by pushing strongly through the thighs and exerting greater effort with the arms.
- Perform the movement with a half turn.
- Perform the movement with a quarter turn and select another movement (Ski Strides) to perform as a transitionary movement before turning back to the original starting position.
- **Neutralise** the movement by starting with the legs straddling the step, and bringing them in and out to touch the step.

## Exercise 9.2 • Ski Jumps (rebounding)

### Purpose

This is a high intensity exercise that should be used specifically in the main workout.

### Starting position and instructions

Stand side-on to the step. Adopt a narrow straddled foot position. Bend the knees and push through the thigh muscles to create an upwards and sideways movement through the water on to the step. The arms should be used to push the water down and away from the desired direction of travel. Repeat the action, jumping from the step to the pool floor, landing at the other side of the step.

### Coaching points

- Keep the knee joint unlocked.
- Ensure the heels go down when landing.
- Ensure the whole foot lands on the step.
- Keep the elbows slightly bent.
- Keep the arms under the water.
- Keep the hips facing forwards.

| **Exercise 9.2** | **Ski Jumps (rebounding)** |
| --- | --- |

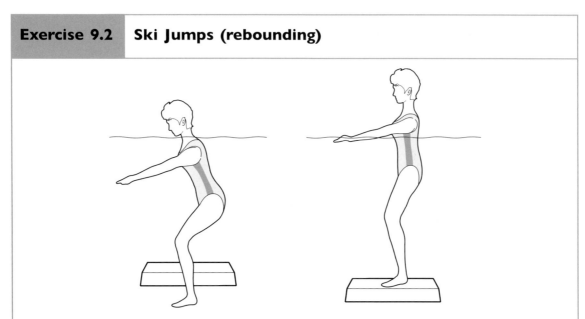

**Choreography note:** Perform a floor-based movement, such as a Spotty Dog, for a number of repetitions before rebounding to the other side.

## Progressions

- Start with a small jump by not pushing forcefully through the thigh muscles.
- Progress to a larger jump and rebound by pushing more forcefully through the thighs.
- Exert greater force with the arms to increase the height of the jump.
- **Neutralise** the movement by starting on top of the step with the knees bent and the body low in the water. Jump the legs to alternate sides of the step, keeping the body low and allowing the feet briefly to touch the step midway through the sequence.
- **Rebound** completely over to the other side of the step.

# Exercise 9.3 • Power Squats (basic)

## Purpose

To elevate and maintain the heart rate.

## Starting position and instructions

Stand on top of the step. Commence by stepping one leg out to the side in a squatting position. The other leg should stay in contact with the step. Push through the thigh, and pull the arms through the water to lift the body back on to the step and into the starting position. Repeat, moving to the other side.

## Coaching points

- Squat the legs to a comfortable range of motion.
- Ensure the knees move in line with the toe and over the ankle.
- Do not let the knees roll inwards.
- Keep the hips facing forwards and avoid hollowing the lower back.
- Avoid locking the knees as the leg straightens.
- Keep the elbows unlocked.

| **Exercise 9.3** | **Power Squats (basic)** |
|---|---|

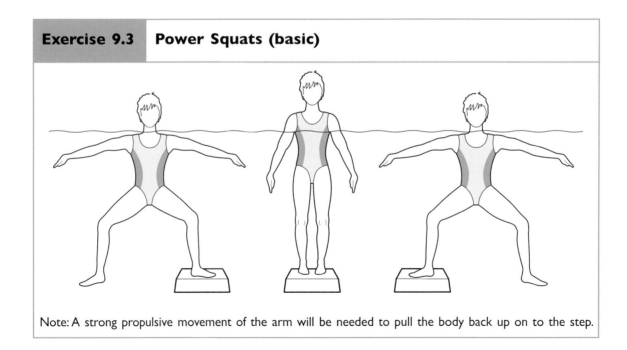

Note: A strong propulsive movement of the arm will be needed to pull the body back up on to the step.

## Progressions

- Start with a small and slow movement.
- Progressively move at a slightly faster pace and make the movement larger.
- Pull more forcefully against the water to return on to the step, and push more forcefully through the thigh.
- **Rebound** the movement by jumping the legs alternately off the step, keeping the body weight over the step, rather than transferring the weight towards the squatting leg.
- **Neutralise** the movement by keeping the body low in the water and jumping the legs as described above for rebounding.

## Exercise 9.4 • Ski Strides (neutral)

### Purpose

To elevate and maintain the heart rate.

## Starting position and instructions

Stand in a straddle foot position, facing the step. Neutralise the body position so that the body stays low in the water. Commence striding the legs alternately backwards and forwards, touching the step lightly with the front foot.

## Coaching points

- Care should be taken not to force the heel of the back leg to the floor, unless it feels comfortable.
- Keep the hips facing forwards.
- Keep the knees and elbows unlocked.

## Progressions

- Start with small strides and increase to a larger range of motion by increasing stride length.
- Move at a progressively faster pace.
- Exert a greater force against the water with the arms and legs.
- Use the arms in opposition to the legs, to assist balance.

| Exercise 9.4 | Ski Strides (neutral) |
|---|---|

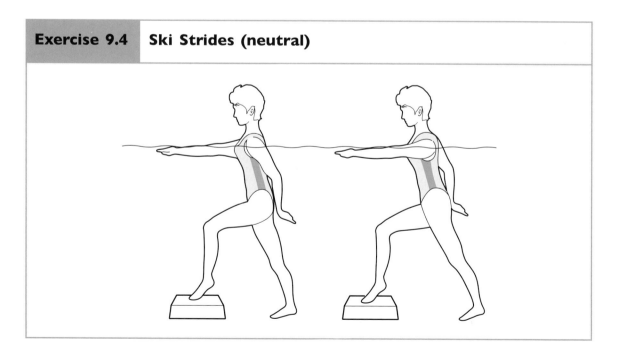

- **Rebound** the movement by lifting the body out of the water on each stride.
- **Suspend** the movement over the step; the feet should not touch the floor or the step.

## Exercise 9.5 • Water Tread (suspended)

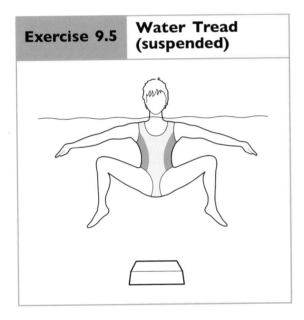

| Exercise 9.5 | **Water Tread (suspended)** |
|---|---|

### Purpose

This exercise will maintain the heart rate.

### Starting position and instructions

Suspend the body over the step so that the legs are not in contact with the pool floor. Use the hands and legs to push the water down and keep the body suspended.

### Coaching points

- Keep the knee joint unlocked.
- Keep the elbows slightly bent and the arms low under the water, level with the hip.
- Keep the hips facing forwards.

### Progressions

- Start with a small pedalling action of the legs and progress to a larger pedalling action.
- Exert a greater force through the thigh and the arms.
- **Neutralise** the movement by keeping the body suspended, but taking the feet lightly to the floor and then up towards the armpits.
- Increase the speed of the movement in a neutral position.

## Exercise 9.6 • Jog Up (basic)

### Purpose

To elevate and maintain the heart rate.

### Starting position

Jog in place. Run up onto the step, pulling the water backwards. Run off the step by pulling the water forwards.

### Coaching points

- Keep the knee joint unlocked.
- Keep the elbows slightly bent.
- Keep the hips facing forwards.
- Ensure the heels go down on landing.

### Progressions

- Start with a light jog onto and off the step.
- Progress by lifting the knees higher and jogging slightly further away from the step.
- Run up at a slightly faster pace.

| Exercise 9.6 | Jog Up (basic) |
| --- | --- |

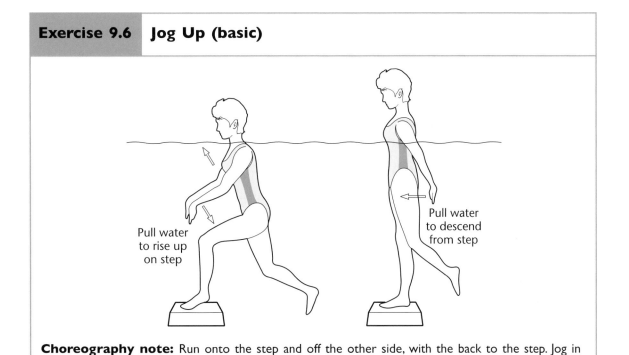

Pull water to rise up on step

Pull water to descend from step

**Choreography note:** Run onto the step and off the other side, with the back to the step. Jog in place. Perform a Sploosh with a half turn and jog in place (16 counts). Repeat the sequence to the other side of the step. (Total 32 counts.)

## Exercise 9.7 • Power Lunges (rebounding)

### Purpose

This exercise will maintain the heart rate.

### Starting position and instructions

Stand side-on to the step with one foot on the step and the other foot on the floor. Push through the thigh of the leg on the step and rebound, lifting the body out of the water so that the body weight moves to the other side of the step and the other foot is now on top of the step. Repeat and return to the starting position. Initially, pull the water towards the body and away from the direction of travel. As the body lifts out of the water, continue to push the water away from the direction of travel.

### Coaching points

- Keep the knee joint unlocked.
- Ensure the foot lands in the centre of the step with each lunge.
- Keep the elbows unlocked.
- Keep the hips facing forwards.

### Progressions

- Start with a small lunge and rebound.
- Progress by rebounding higher.
- Move at a slightly faster pace.
- **Neutralise** the movement by keeping the body low and under the water, and lightly tapping the step with the feet.

| Exercise 9.7 | Power Lunges (rebounding) |
|---|---|

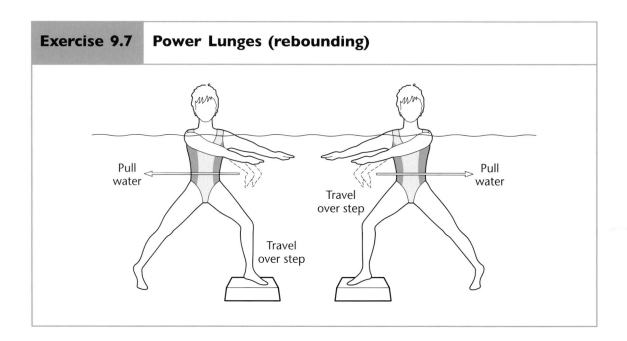

# DESIGNING A MUSCULAR STRENGTH AND ENDURANCE TRAINING PROGRAMME

10

## OBJECTIVES

By the end of this chapter the reader will be able to:

* Recognise a safe and effective structure to improve muscular fitness in a water-based session
* Identify a range of factors that will affect the timing, intensity, structure and content of the muscular strength and endurance (MSE) component in a water-based session
* Recognise a range of safe and effective exercises for inclusion in the MSE component or within an MSE training session
* Describe the effects of water on MSE training
* Describe different methods of MSE training that can be adapted for use in a water-based session
* Recognise methods of adapting the exercises to cater for different levels of ability and fitness.

Specific muscular strength and endurance activities can be included as a secondary main workout in most programmes. An appropriate session structure is shown in table 8.1, page 125. However, it is also possible to devote a whole session to these two components of fitness. An appropriate structure for this specific type of programme is outlined in table 10.1, page 154.

This chapter provides guidelines for structuring the muscular strength and endurance component, whether as a secondary or main workout. It also illustrates exercises for the major muscle groups. The benefits of training to improve muscular strength and endurance are discussed in Chapter 2.

## What activities are appropriate to improve muscular strength and endurance?

Activities that require the muscles to contract and work through a full range of motion are appropriate. Some appropriate exercises are outlined in table 10.2, page 157; others are illustrated at the end of this chapter. To improve muscular endurance, it will be necessary to work the muscles for longer (higher repetitions) with less resistance to movement. To improve muscular strength, it will be necessary to create further resistance to movement so that fewer repetitions of the activity can be performed.

| **Table 10.1** | **Session structure for a muscular strength and endurance session** |
|---|---|

**Warm-up**
- Mobility and pulse-raising activities
- Preparatory stretches
- Re-warm

**Muscular strength and endurance training**
- Specific toning exercises targeting all major muscle groups to achieve a balanced, whole body approach

**Cool-down**
- Cooling down exercises
- Post-workout stretches
- Relaxation activities (optional)
- Re-mobilise.

**Note:** it is safe and effective to include cardiovascular training exercises between toning work. However, the intensity of the re-warmer will need to be increased to a slightly higher level. The intensity of the cool-down will also need to start at a slightly higher intensity.

Note: If a cardiovascular training component precedes muscular strength and endurance training then it may not be necessary to target certain muscles again. The muscles not used in the preceding component should be prioritised.

Water provides a natural resistance to all movements. The muscles will have to work harder to overcome this resistance. The added resistance may well be sufficient to challenge a less fit group and improve their muscular strength. However, for most people, the resistance will be relatively easy to overcome and most improvements will be for muscular endurance. To add further resistance and challenge a fitter group, buoyancy equipment can be used to increase the surface area and drag. Working with longer levers, and moving at a slightly faster pace, will also make the activities more intense.

## NEED TO KNOW

**Summary of training to improve muscular strength and endurance**

To improve muscular endurance – perform more repetitions.

To improve muscular strength – create further resistance to movement. Add resistance by:

- increasing the range of motion
- increasing the speed of the exercise
- increasing the surface area moved
- increasing the leverage.

Make the component harder by:

- increasing the component time
- including more exercises
- working the same muscle a few times (multiple sets)
- working more muscles.

**Note:** whether strength or endurance is improved will depend on the number of repetitions one is able to perform.

Lower rep ranges (1–10) will primarily improve strength.

Higher rep ranges (15–30) will primarily improve endurance.

Mid rep ranges (8–15) will improve muscular fitness.

## How will exercising in water affect the component structure?

Water provides a constant and multi-dimensional resistance to all movements. The muscles will contract differently when moving in water. Most of the eccentric muscle work will be eliminated and the majority of muscular contractions will be dual-concentric, the exception being exercises using buoyancy equipment to add resistance (discussed in Chapter 1). A greater number of muscles will be working to perform a specific exercise, so exercising the muscles in water will potentially provide a more balanced approach.

## NEED TO KNOW

- Concentric – shortening of the muscle to create movement against a resistance (e.g. when lifting against the force of gravity on land).
- Eccentric – lengthening of the muscle to control movement yielding against a resistance (e.g. when lowering against the force of gravity on land).
- Isometric – static contraction of the muscle to hold a position without movement.

**In water:**

- Most muscle work will be concentric because the body movement is resisted in all directions.
- There will be high demands on fixating the trunk (isometric work) to maintain balance in water. This will improve core stability.
- When equipment devices are used, there may be some eccentric work – e.g. a water bell (when under water) will pull towards flotation to the water surface. To control this flotation, the muscle contraction would be eccentric.

The temperature of the water will have a cooling effect on the body. Therefore, to keep warm it will be necessary to perform some larger pulse-raising exercises between muscular strength and endurance exercises. Alternating upper and lower body work is another effective way of maintaining a comfortable temperature.

The buoyancy of the water will require the exercise positions to be selected carefully to ensure that the body remains stable. It may be necessary to perform propulsive movements of the arms to keep the position stable and prevent loss of balance.

---

### NEED TO KNOW

- MSE exercises need to be dynamic and constant to maintain body temperature and prevent cooling.
- Any part of the body that is out of the water may chill.

---

## Muscular resistance training approaches and systems

There are different approaches to traditional gym-based resistance training that can be adapted for use in a water-based session to add variety and achieve specific fitness goals.

### Super sets/Giant sets

This approach is used in gym-based sessions by bodybuilders to increase muscular size and growth – hypertrophy (Fleck and Kraemer, 1987:91). There are two methods of super setting; both methods involve continuous movement from one exercise to the next without rest. Usually, 8-10 repetitions of each exercise are performed in the gym-based environment.

### Method one

Involves working the prime mover/agonist and then the antagonist muscle.
Land example: super set
- Bicep Curls
- Tricep Kick Backs

The issue with using this approach in an exercise in water session is that the majority of muscle work in water is dual-concentric and therefore follows a super setting approach. For example: Bear Hugs illustrated on page 170, performed in water, work both the pectorals and trapezius muscles.

However, using equipment in the session and against the buoyancy of the water can change the muscle work and may bring about single muscle work, and both concentric and eccentric contractions.

| Table 10.2 | Joint actions when the major muscle groups contract concentrically | | | |
|---|---|---|---|---|
| Muscle name | Anatomical position | Joints crossed | Prime action when contracting concentrically | Exercise |
| Gastrocnemius | Calf muscle | Knee and ankle | Plantar flexion – pointing the toe | Rising on to the ball of the foot |
| Soleus | Calf muscle | Ankle | As above – with knee bent | As above – with knee bent |
| Tibialis anterior | Front of shin bone | Ankle | Dorsi flexion of the ankle | Toe tapping |
| Hamstrings | Back of thigh | Knee and hip | Flexion of the knee | Lifting the heel towards the buttocks |
| Quadriceps | Front of thigh | Knee and hip | Extension of the knee | Straightening the knee (squats) |
| Gluteus maximus | Buttock | Hip | Extension of the hip | Lifting the leg out straight behind the body |
| Iliopsoas (hip flexor) | Front hip | Hip | Flexion of the hip | Lifting knees to the chest |
| Abductors | Outside of hip and thigh | Hip | Abduction of the leg | Taking the leg out to the side of the body |
| Adductors | Inside thigh | Hip | Adduction of the hip | Taking the leg across the front of the body |
| Rectus abdominus | Abdominals (front) | Spine | Flexion of the spine | Bending the spine forwards |
| Erector spinae | Back of spine | Spine | Extension of the spine | Straightening the spine |

| Table 10.2 | Joint actions when the major muscle groups contract concentrically (cont.) | | | |
|---|---|---|---|---|
| Muscle name | Anatomical position | Joints crossed | Prime action when contracting concentrically | Exercise |
| Obliques | Side of trunk | Spine | Lateral flexion and rotation of the spine | Twisting and bending the trunk to the side |
| Pectorals | Front of chest | Shoulder | Adduction and horizontal flexion of the arm | Bringing the arms across the front of the body (Bear Hug) |
| Trapezius | Upper and middle back | Shoulder girdle | Extension of the neck | Keeping the head up |
| | | | Elevation of the shoulder | Lifting and lowering the shoulders |
| | | | Retraction of the scapula | Squeezing the shoulder blades together |
| Latissimus dorsi | Side of back | Shoulder | Adduction of the shoulder | Drawing the arms across the body |
| Deltoids | Top of the shoulder | Shoulder | Abduction of the shoulder | Lifting the arms out to the side |
| Biceps | Front of the upper arm | Elbow and shoulder | Flexion of the elbow | Bending the elbow |
| Triceps | Back of the upper arm | Elbow and shoulder | Extension of the elbow | Straightening the elbow (press-ups) |

NB: This table provides a basic introduction to muscle actions. Persons interested in reading further are referred to other references listed at the back of this book.

> **For example:**
> Using an elbow curl action with water bells: the triceps will work eccentrically to raise the water bells to the surface, and concentrically to lower the water bells down through the water against buoyancy. In this instance, another exercise for the opposite muscle can be found to super set with the tricep exercise described.

## Method two

Involves performing a number of different exercises for the same muscle group in succession. This is sometimes referred to as giant sets or compound/tri-sets. In water, three different exercises for the same body areas can be used to create a water-based giant set.

For example: **ONE** giant set
- Mermaids – page 161
- Twisters – page 162
- Sweep Through – page 163

The benefits of using the super or giant sets method are that it enables continuous muscle work, which potentially enables the work time to be reduced. A further advantage, in water, is that constant movement helps to keep the body warm. The disadvantage would be that super/giant setting demands a good base level of fitness to manage the constant workload/resistance. However, in water, the resistance can be adapted by manipulating the surface area and also the equipment. These variables will also change the intensity of the exercises.

## Pyramids

Pyramid or triangle programmes are used in gym-based programmes, predominantly by power lifters. A full pyramid would start with a low resistance for 10–12 repetitions. This would develop over a number of sets by performing less repetitions and a heavier resistance to a level where a maximum of one repetition would be performed in a true pyramid. The process would then be reversed altering the same variables to lower the resistance and increase the repetitions.

Water naturally adds resistance to the movements performed, however, it is unlikely that the resistance would be sufficient enough to achieve a one repetition maximum level (one rep max = most resistance that can be lifted once by a muscle or muscle group).

Pyramid training can still be modified for use in water, by manipulating the variables that do exist to increase resistance to movement: surface area, speed of movement, force exerted, and equipment.

### Example pyramid within water-based session – varying speed

15 repetitions – Bear Hugs – slower pace
10 repetitions – Bear Hugs – stronger force
 6 repetitions – Bear Hugs – as fast as possible
10 repetitions – Bear Hugs – stronger force
15 repetitions – Bear Hugs – slower pace

### Example pyramid within water-based session – varying surface area

10 reps – elbow extension with water mitts
 8 reps – elbow extension with water bells – narrow edge leads
 6 reps – elbow extension with water bells – wide edge leads
 8 reps – elbow extension with water bells – narrow edge leads
10 reps – elbow extension with water mitts

Vary this method by only performing the ascending first half of the pyramid/triangle (low to high workload) or only performing the descending half of the pyramid/triangle (high to low workload).

## SHORT ANSWER REVISION QUESTIONS

1 Name **TWO** components that are essential for inclusion in any programme.

2 Which component (strength or endurance) would be trained most in an exercise in water session? Give reasons for your answer.

3 Describe how exercise in water may improve core stability.

4 Describe how temperature may affect the MSE component.

5 Describe how frontal resistance will affect muscle contraction in water.

6 Describe how using buoyancy equipment may affect some exercises in water.

7 Describe how super and giant sets can be adapted for use in a water-based session.

8 Describe how pyramid training can be adapted for use in a water-based session.

# Resistance exercises to improve muscular strength and endurance

## Exercise 10.1 • Mermaids

### Purpose

This exercise will work the abdominal muscles at the front and side of the trunk (the rectus abdominus and obliques).

### Starting position and instructions

Use a float or tube to maintain flotation. Float the legs to one side of the body. Contract the abdominal muscles and bend the knees towards the chest. Drag the body sideways through the water, and extend the legs. The legs should be floating at the other side of the body. Repeat, dragging the legs through the water and back to their initial starting position.

### Coaching points

• Tighten the abdominal muscles.
• Initiate the movement by moving the trunk of the body.
• Take care not to hollow the back.

### Progressions

• Start with a slow movement and progressively increase the speed.
• Perform the exercise holding on to poolside.
• Perform the exercise free-floating, using a sculling movement of the arm to maintain flotation.
• Use ankle cuffs and water bells to increase surface area and drag through the water.

| Exercise 10.1 | Mermaids |
| --- | --- |

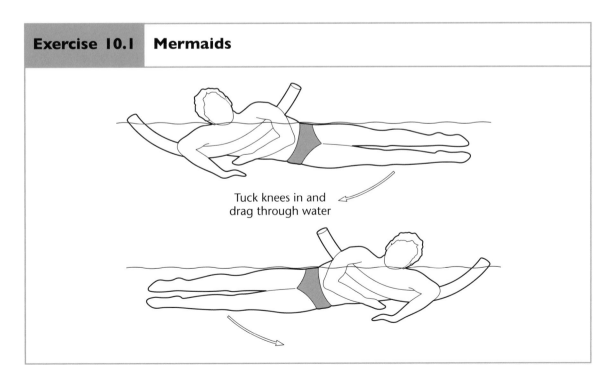

Tuck knees in and drag through water

## Exercise 10.2 • Twisters

### Purpose

This exercise will work muscles at the front and side of the trunk (rectus abdominus and obliques).

### Starting position and instructions

Lift the knees towards the chest and suspend the body in the water by using floats under each arm. Twist the knees towards one side and then back to the centre. Repeat to the other side.

### Coaching points

- Initiate the movement from the abdominals.
- Pull the abdominals in tight.
- Rotate from the middle of the trunk.
- Take care not to twist the lower back.

### Progressions

- Start slowly and progress by moving at a slightly faster pace.

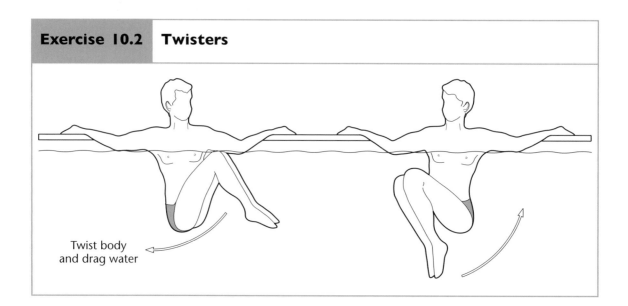

**Exercise 10.2**    **Twisters**

Twist body
and drag water

## Exercise 10.3 • Sweep Through

### Purpose

This exercise will work muscles at the front and side of the trunk (rectus abdominus and obliques).

### Starting position and instructions

Lie on the front of the body and hold the poolside. It is easier to maintain flotation if one hand holds the rail and the other hand is positioned about a foot below, against the poolside. Contract the abdominal muscles and bend the knees towards the chest. Drag the legs through the water, until the feet can touch the pool wall.

Contract the abdominals again and reverse the movement. Extend the legs once the buttocks are close to the surface of the water.

### Coaching points

- Ensure the lower back does not hollow as the legs return to the water surface.
- Keep the movement controlled.
- Keep the abdominals pulled in.
- Keep the head in line with the spine.

### Progressions

- Perform with floats or a tube and fully extend the legs so that the body is lying backwards in the water to increase the range of motion. (This combines movement of Float and Pull exercise, illustrated next.)
- Perform free-floating, using sculling movements of the arms to maintain flotation.

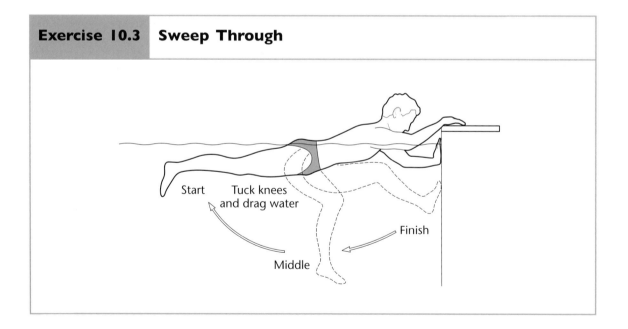

| Exercise 10.3 | Sweep Through |
|---|---|

## Exercise 10.4 • Float and Pull

### Purpose

This exercise will work the muscles at the front and side of the trunk (the rectus abdominus and obliques).

### Starting position and instructions

Lie with the back to the pool surface and hold the poolside (alternative grips are illustrated in Chapter 1). Allow the legs to float upwards towards the surface of the water. Contract the abdominal muscles and pull the buttocks down through the water towards the pool wall. Repeat the movement.

### Coaching points

- Take care not to hollow the back as the legs rise to the water surface.
- Pull in the abdominals.
- Relax the shoulders.

### Progressions

- Perform the exercise slowly and progress to performing it slightly faster.
- Use a buoyancy belt around hips to increase the resistance.
- Combine with Sweep Through exercise and perform in the middle of the pool with either a float, a tube, or free-floating in the middle of the pool. Note: strong propulsive movements of the arm will be needed to assist the movement and maintain flotation.

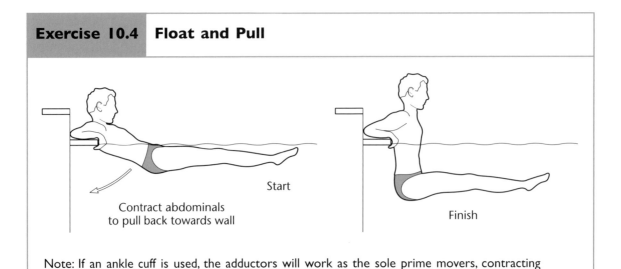

**Exercise 10.4** | **Float and Pull**

Contract abdominals to pull back towards wall

Start

Finish

Note: If an ankle cuff is used, the adductors will work as the sole prime movers, contracting eccentrically as the leg lifts to the surface of the water, and concentrically to pull the leg down through the water and slightly across the body.

## Exercise 10.5 • Side Leg Raises

### Purpose

This exercise will work the muscles on the inside and outside of the thigh (the adductors and abductors).

### Starting position and instructions

Stand facing the pool and hold on to the pool-side. Lift the leg out to the side of the body and towards the surface of the water. Pull the leg back down through the water and take it slightly across the front of the body.

### Coaching points

- Keep the supporting knee joint slightly bent and do not allow the knee to roll in.
- Only raise the leg to a comfortable height. Do not allow the hip to rotate outward and roll back.
- Keep the hips facing forwards.
- Keep a space between the hips and ribcage.
- Drag the side of the foot through the water.
- Keep the body upright.

### Progressions

- Work initially through a small range of motion and at a slow pace.
- Progress to lifting the leg higher and working at a faster pace.
- Use an ankle cuff or water fins for added resistance.

**Exercise 10.5** **Side Leg Raises**

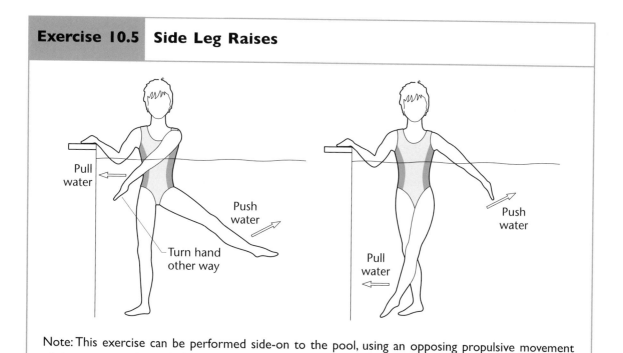

Note: This exercise can be performed side-on to the pool, using an opposing propulsive movement of the arm to maintain balance and correct posture.

# Exercise 10.6 • Scissor Legs

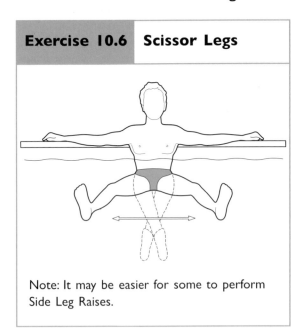

| Exercise 10.6 | Scissor Legs |
| --- | --- |

Note: It may be easier for some to perform Side Leg Raises.

## Coaching points

- Keep the knees unlocked.
- Keep the hips square.
- Maintain the natural curve of the lower back, but do not allow the back to hollow.

## Progressions

- Start slowly; progress by increasing the speed.
- Vary the tempo: two slow and four quick.
- Use ankle cuffs or fins to increase surface area and, therefore, resistance.
- Perform in the middle of the pool using a tube, floats or buoyancy belt.

## Purpose

This exercise will work the muscles on the inside and outside of the thigh and hip (the adductors and the abductors).

## Starting position and instructions

Lie with the back or front to the pool, holding the poolside. Allow the legs to float upwards to a level that is comfortable. The legs can stay low if it is more comfortable. Take the legs apart as far as is comfortable, then draw them together and scissor one across the other.

## Exercise 10.7 • Leg Extensions

### Purpose

To work the buttock muscles (gluteals).

### Starting position and instructions

Stand facing the pool and hold on to the poolside. Lift the leg in front of the body and level with the hip. Contract the muscles of the buttocks (gluteals) and press the leg down through the water. Take the leg further back from the original starting position to increase the range of motion. Return the leg to the original position.

### Coaching points

- Ensure the lower back does not hollow.
- Pull in the abdominals.
- Do not take the leg too far back.
- Keep the hips facing forwards.
- Keep the supporting knee joint unlocked.

### Progressions

- Start at a slow pace and progress by working at a faster pace.
- Start with a bent knee and progress to performing the exercise with a straight leg.
- Progress by adding ankle cuffs or water fins to the ankle to increase the surface area.
- Perform in deeper water with a buoyancy aid, using both legs in opposition by performing Spotty Dogs, illustrated on page 100.

| Exercise 10.7 | Leg Extensions |
| --- | --- |

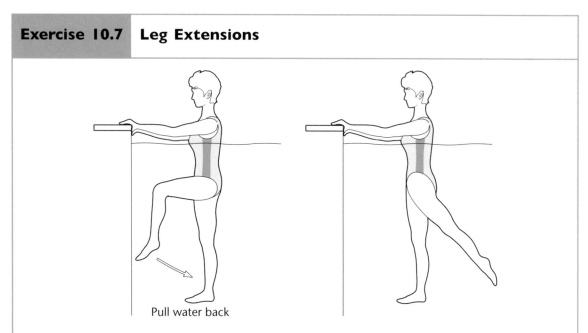

Pull water back

Note: It will be necessary to perform this exercise side-on to the pool if a full lever is used. An opposing propulsive movement of the arm will be necessary to maintain balance and correct posture.

## Exercise 10.8 • Flip Flaps

### Purpose

This exercise will work the muscles at the front and back of the hip and thigh (the hip flexors, quadriceps, gluteals and hamstrings).

### Starting position and instructions

Lie on the front facing the pool surface and hold the poolside. Pull one leg down through the water so that the toes rest on the floor: the other leg should be at the surface of the water. Drag the other leg down through the water and push the opposite leg to the surface to change leg positions. Repeat.

### Coaching points

- Ensure the lower back does not hollow.
- Keep the knee joints unlocked.
- Keep the hips square so that the lower spine does not twist.

### Progressions

- Start with short levers by bending the knees, and progress to the longer levers.
- Start with a small range of motion by not taking the leg so far down to the floor. Progress to working through a fuller range of motion.
- Progress by increasing the speed.
- Vary the tempo and range of motion. Perform eight slowly and through a full range of motion, and 16 quickly through a smaller range of motion by splashing the legs at the surface of the water.

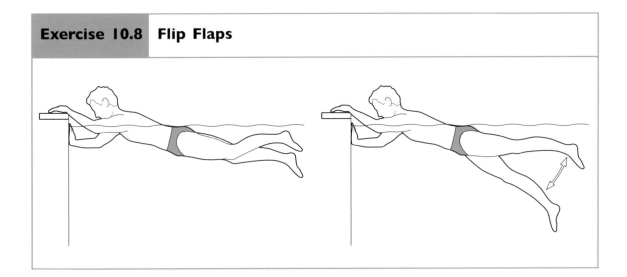

**Exercise 10.8    Flip Flaps**

## Exercise 10.9 • Pool Press-ups

### Purpose

This exercise will work the muscles at the front of the chest and shoulder (the pectorals and anterior deltoid). It will also work the muscles at the back of the upper arm (the triceps).

### Starting position and instructions

Place the hands on the poolside or hold on to the gully. Lift the body out of the water by pushing through the arms, and fully straighten the elbows. Lower the body, under control, back down through the water.

### Coaching points

- Keep the shoulders level and press evenly through both arms to lift the bodyweight out of the water.

- Ensure the elbows do not lock.
- Keep the back straight.

### Progressions

- If the exercise is too hard, start by holding the gully or pool rail with the feet on the floor. Pull the body towards the rail and push the body away from the rail. Build up the repetitions performed for this exercise before progressing.
- Use the feet to push from the pool floor to assist the arms lifting the bodyweight out of the water.
- Initially work through a small range of motion by lifting the body out as far as possible, and then returning to the water.
- Progress by moving more slowly. This exercise utilises gravity as a resistance, so performing faster will be easier.

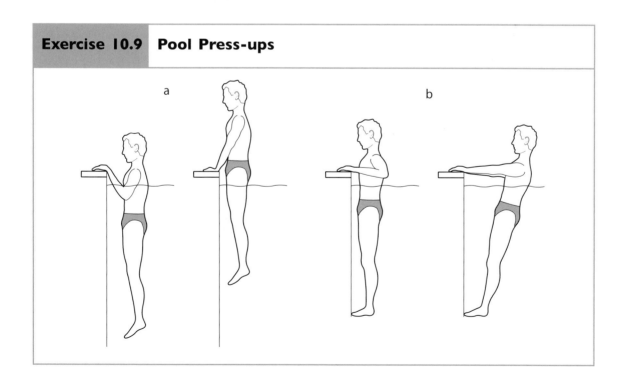

| Exercise 10.9 | Pool Press-ups |
|---|---|

## Exercise 10.10 • Bear Hugs

### Purpose

This exercise will work the muscles at the front of the chest (the pectorals) and the muscles of the middle back (the trapezius).

### Starting position and instructions

Adopt a staggered or straddle foot stance. Allow the arms to lift to the surface of the water. Contract the muscles of the chest and drag the arms through the water and in front of the body, crossing over slightly. To return, contract the muscles in between the shoulder blades and drag the arms back through the water and behind the body, as far as is comfortable. Repeat.

### Coaching points

- Keep the knees unlocked.
- Keep the hips facing forwards.
- Keep the elbows unlocked.
- Keep the arms under water.
- Pull in the abdominals.

### Progressions

- Start by moving through a small range of motion and by exerting only a little force against the water.
- Progress by moving through a larger range of motion, moving at a slightly faster pace, and exerting more force against the water in both directions.
- Progress further by using mitts, floats, water bells or a tube to increase the surface area.

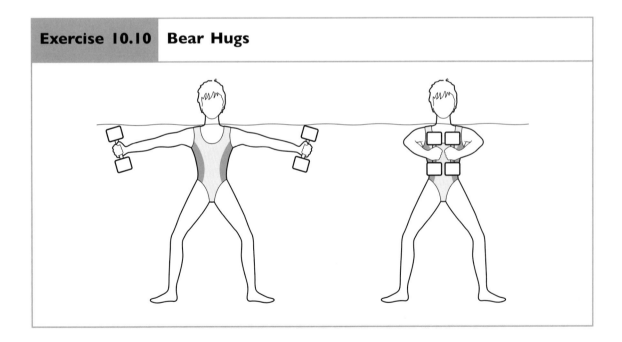

| Exercise 10.10 | Bear Hugs |
|---|---|

## Exercise 10.11 • Elbow Extensions (using a tube or delta bells)

| Exercise 10.11 | Elbow Extensions |
|---|---|

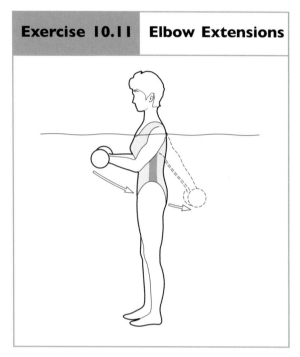

### Purpose

This exercise will work the triceps muscles at the back of the upper arm.

### Starting position and instructions

Adopt a comfortable and stable foot position. Keep the elbows in to the sides of the body. Hold the water bells or tube with an overhand grip, and allow them to float at the water surface. Commence the exercise by pressing the arms down through the water and fully extending the elbow. Return the arms to the surface with control. (This will maximise the eccentric contraction required from the muscle to return the device to the surface.)

### Coaching points

- Keep the elbows tight to the sides.
- Fully extend, but do not lock the elbows.
- Keep the knees unlocked.
- Control the return movement of the arms to the water surface.
- Keep the back straight.

### Progressions

- Start with no equipment, or just water mitts, and work at a slower pace.
- Progress to using devices that increase flotation of the limbs (tubes and water bells).
- If necessary, start by working through a small range of motion (halfway down). Progress to working through a full range of motion and at a slightly faster pace.

# SHORT ANSWER REVISION QUESTIONS

State **ONE** exercise that will work the following muscles in water and describe the muscle contraction:

| Muscle | Exercise | Muscle contraction |
| --- | --- | --- |
| Bicep | | |
| Tricep | | |
| Adductors | | |
| Abductors | | |
| Gluteals | | |
| Quadriceps | | |
| Hamstrings | | |
| Pectorals | | |
| Trapezius | | |

# USING SPECIALIST EQUIPMENT AND DEEP-WATER TRAINING

11

## OBJECTIVES

By the end of this chapter the reader will be able to:

- Recognise a range of equipment that can be used in an exercise in water session
- Recognise a range of exercises using equipment
- State some of the advantages and disadvantages of using equipment in a water-based session
- Describe some of the ways different equipment can be used (flotation and/or intensity)
- State some benefits of deep-water training
- State some safety considerations for deep-water training
- Recognise how exercising in deeper water increases the effects of water on the body.

There is a whole range of buoyancy and flotation equipment available. This chapter identifies how it can be used in a session.

## Why use equipment?

Equipment can be used in any session and may serve a number of purposes. It may:

- add variety and interest
- motivate participants and promote further adherence to the programme
- add intensity to cardiovascular and muscular strength and endurance activities
- provide a progression to the programme of activities
- be used to assist rehabilitation of injuries (only by physiotherapists in latter stages)
- provide an excellent method for multi-level groups when used in a circuit training session.

However, because most equipment will intensify the workout, it is advisable to:

- only use equipment if participants are capable, and of an appropriate skill and fitness level
- progress gradually, starting with slower movements and shorter levers if possible, or using a smaller surface area of the equipment under the water
- maintain correct posture and joint alignment: do not lock out the joints
- ensure a balanced approach (work opposing muscles)
- keep equipment under the water (unless using water bells half out of the water to minimise intensity)
- wash equipment after use.

# What equipment is available?

The wide range of equipment available includes:
- buoyancy belts and belt hitch
- tubes/woggles
- water bells and ankle cuffs
- mitts and gloves
- steps
- aqua boots and wet vests
- circuit training cards.

## Buoyancy belts and belt hitch

These are primarily used during deep-water programmes to assist flotation and perform cardiovascular training activities. However, they can be used in shallower water to provide greater buoyancy and reduce impact stress for leaner or muscular body types, specialist groups, or those recovering from injuries.

They are excellent for working with runners and other sportspeople. A belt hitch that attaches

**Fig. 11.1 Buoyancy belt and belt hitch**

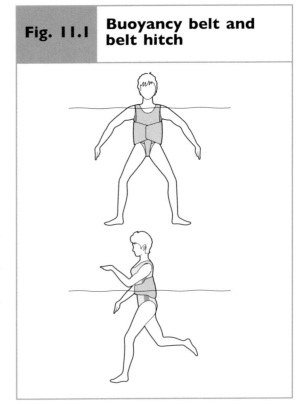

**Fig. 11.2 Tube (or woggle)**

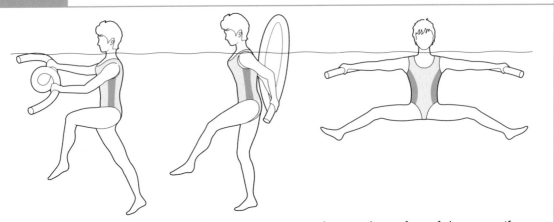

Note: Care must be taken when using buoyancy equipment close to the surface of the water; if movements are not controlled, and/or if too many repetitions are performed, the muscles around the shoulder girdle may be overused and injury may occur.

from the belt to poolside can be used to prevent travel around the pool.

Some designs of buoyancy belt tend to move and ride up the body and can be uncomfortable for women with a large bust. They are fairly expensive to purchase, but are a worthwhile investment for teachers and instructors who personally train clients in water.

## Tubes or woggles

Tubes or woggles are available in most centres offering water-based programmes. They can be used relatively easily and safely by most participants and for many purposes. They are comparatively inexpensive and are useful for:

- assisting flotation to perform suspended activities
- assisting flotation in relaxation activities
- adding intensity to muscular strength and endurance exercises
- adding intensity to some cardiovascular training sessions
- adding fun to the session.

## Water bells and ankle cuffs

Participants need to be confident in water and of a reasonable fitness level to use bells and cuffs together in water.

Prices vary, however this equipment is very useable and therefore a worthwhile investment. Combined use of bells and cuffs will intensify cardiovascular training activities and provide excellent resistance to all movements. Use of water bells on their own is an excellent way of adding resistance to muscular strength and endurance exercises. They are also useful for instructors and teachers who work with personal training clients.

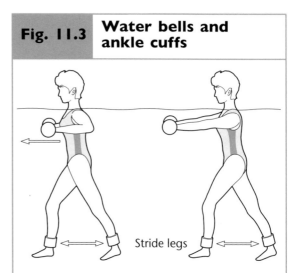

**Fig. 11.3 Water bells and ankle cuffs**

Stride legs

Note: Ankle cuffs should not be worn without holding a water bell, otherwise the legs will rise out of the water and the trunk will be forced under the water from changes in buoyancy.

## Mitts and gloves

Webbed gloves or mitts fit tightly to the hands and will increase the resistance to upper body movements. They can be used by most participants and will assist the performance of propulsive movements. They are useful in most sessions; they can be used in the cardiovascular component to assist with pull against the water

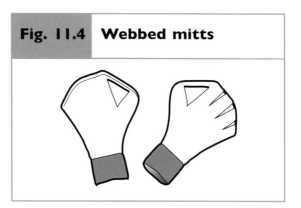

**Fig. 11.4 Webbed mitts**

and are excellent for assisting movements during a step training session. For fitter groups they can be used in the warm-up.

## Steps

Steps tend to be expensive and few centres in the UK have sufficient numbers to hold a large class. However, they provide an interesting and effective circuit training station so it is useful to have access to a few steps. Most of the steps manufactured for use in water tend to move and travel slightly: time can be wasted trying to keep the step in place! Care also needs to be taken not to move the joints out of alignment.

## Floats

Floats are available in all pools and can be used for a number of purposes. These include:
- increasing the intensity of upper body work
- assisting flotation for deep-water activities
- assisting flotation for some muscular strength and endurance exercises
- assisting flotation for relaxation activities.

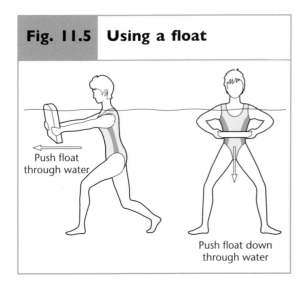

**Fig. 11.5   Using a float**

Push float through water

Push float down through water

## Aqua boots and wet vests

Aqua boots assist traction and protect the feet. They are very useful when working in pools with either a slippery or scratchy floor surface.

Wet vests help to keep the upper body warm and are useful in cooler pools. They are also good for shallow water walking or toning programmes where the upper body may be positioned out of the water for a period of time.

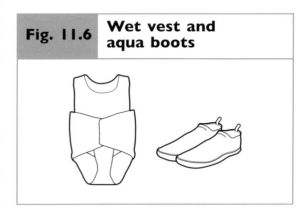

**Fig. 11.6   Wet vest and aqua boots**

## Home-made equipment

Although it is advisable to use equipment that is specifically manufactured for use in the pool, some equipment can be made from household objects. Frisbees, water jugs and washing-up liquid bottles can all be used to add resistance to muscular strength and endurance activities.

If any equipment is used in the session, care should be taken to ensure the moving joints maintain the correct alignment. Equipment should only be used if the participant has sufficient skill to maintain this alignment. The instructor will need to be more attentive when equipment is used to ensure correct technique is maintained.

In Fig. 11.7: (1) Exercise the buttocks and legs by placing the foot on top of the frisbee and pushing down through the water. (Use the wall for balance.)

**Fig. 11.7   Frisbees**

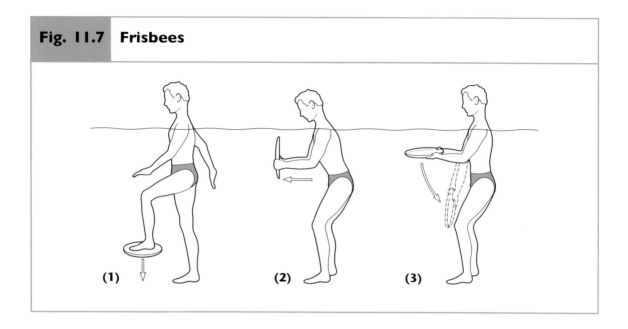

(2) Exercise the upper body by pushing the frisbee through the water with both hands (chest and back) or (3) by pushing the frisbee down through the water for Elbow Extensions (triceps).

In Fig. 11.8: Use the water jug to drag through the water and add intensity to (1) Bear Hugs and (2) Elbow Extensions. Use the washing-up liquid bottles to press sideways and down through the water (3) to exercise muscles at the side of the back.

**Fig. 11.8   Plastic water jug/washing-up liquid bottle**

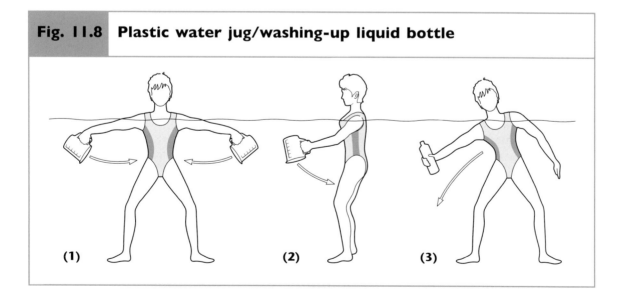

# Exercises using equipment

## Exercise 11.1 • Chest and Back Press (using a tube or delta bells)

| Exercise 11.1 | Chest and Back Press (using a tube or delta bells) |
|---|---|

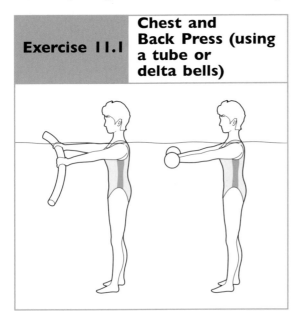

### Purpose

This exercise will work the triceps muscles at the back of the upper arm and pectoral muscles at the front of the chest when pushing forwards, and the biceps muscle (front of upper arm) and latissmus dorsi and trapezius (back muscles) when pulling backwards.

### Starting position and instructions

Adopt a comfortable and stable foot position. Hold the water bells or tube with an overhand grip, and allow them to float at the water surface. Start pressing the equipment forwards and backwards through the water, fully extending the elbow.

### Coaching points

- Keep the abdominals pulled in.
- Keep the shoulders relaxed and down.
- Fully extend, but do not lock the elbows.
- Keep the knees unlocked.
- Keep the back straight.

### Progressions

- If using water bells or paddles, allow half of the equipment to stay out of the water, reducing the surface area.
- Work at a slower pace.
- Work through a smaller range of motion.
- Progress to working through a full range of motion and at a slightly faster pace.

## Exercise 11.2 • Leg Press (with woggle/tube)

| Exercise 11.2 | Leg Press (with woggle/tube) |
|---|---|

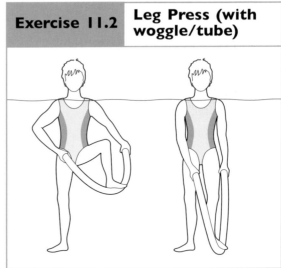

### Purpose

This exercise will work the gluteal muscles (buttocks), hamstrings (back thigh) and quadriceps (front thigh).

### Starting position and instructions

Adopt a comfortable and stable foot position. Hold one end of the woggle in each hand and place a foot in the centre of the woggle. Press the woggle down through the water, fully extending the knee and hip.

## Coaching points

- Keep the abdominals pulled in.
- Keep the shoulders relaxed and down.
- Fully extend, but do not lock the knees.
- Keep the support knee unlocked.
- Keep the back straight.

## Progressions

- Work at a slower pace.
- Work through a smaller range of motion.
- Progress to working through a full range of motion and at a slightly faster pace.
- Place back against pool wall to assist balance.

## Exercise 11.3 • Partner Pull

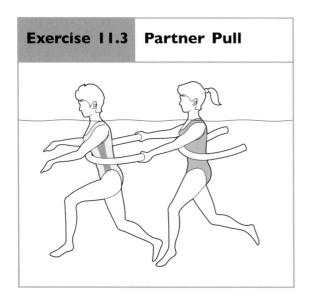

**Exercise 11.3 | Partner Pull**

## Purpose

This exercise can be used in the cardiovascular component to add resistance to running.

## Starting position and instructions

Each partner places a woggle around their waist. One partner stands behind the other and holds the ends of the partner's woggle. Both partners run through the water. The partner at the back pulls on the woggle to add resistance.

## Coaching points:

- Keep the abdominals pulled in.
- Ensure the shoulders are relaxed and down.
- Keep the knees and elbows unlocked.
- Keep the back straight.

## Progressions

- Work at a slower pace.
- Pull lightly on partner's woggle.
- Increase pace and add more resistance by pulling harder on partner's woggle or tube.

## Exercise 11.4 • Chest and Back Squeeze (with woggle)

### Purpose

**Front squeeze:** This exercise will work the pectoral muscles (at the front of the chest).
**Back squeeze:** This exercise will work the latissimus dorsi and trapezius muscles (the side and the middle back).

### Starting position and instructions

Adopt a comfortable and stable foot position. Hold an end of the woggle in each hand. Hold the woggle either in front of or behind the body, and squeeze the ends of the woggle together.

### Coaching points

* Keep the abdominals pulled in.
* Keep the shoulders relaxed and down.
* Fully extend, but do not lock the elbows.
* Keep the back straight.

### Progressions

* Work at a slower pace.
* Work through a smaller range of motion.
* Progress to working through a full range of motion and at a slightly faster pace.
* Combine with a Jumping Jack leg movement (see page 137).

| Exercise 11.4 | Chest and Back Squeeze (with woggle) |
|---|---|

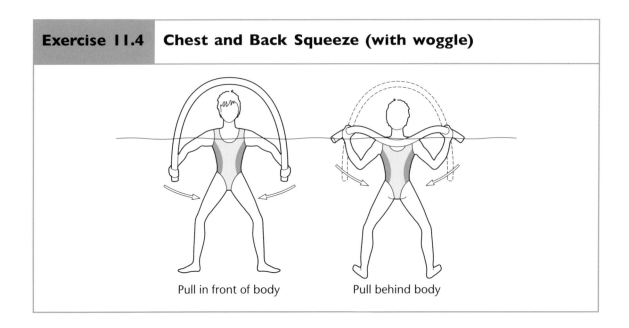

Pull in front of body          Pull behind body

## Exercise 11.5 • Chest and Rotator Cuff (with woggle)

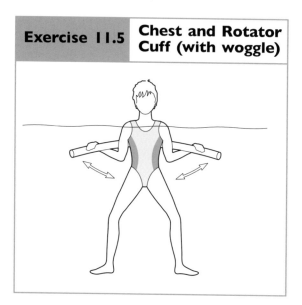

| Exercise 11.5 | Chest and Rotator Cuff (with woggle) |
|---|---|

### Purpose

**Front squeeze**: This exercise will work the pectoral muscles (at the front of the chest).
**Back squeeze**: This exercise will work the muscles at the shoulder girdle (the rotator cuff).

### Starting position and instructions

Adopt a comfortable and stable foot position. Place the woggle around the waist and hold one end in each hand with the elbows close to the sides of the body throughout. Squeeze the ends of the woggle together in front of the body. Rotate the forearm outwards and push the ends of the woggle away from each other.

### Coaching points

- Keep the abdominals pulled in.
- Keep the shoulders relaxed and down.
- Keep the elbows close to the body.
- Keep the back straight.
- Make sure the knees are unlocked.

### Progressions

- Work at a slower pace.
- Work through a smaller range of motion.
- Progress to working through a full range of motion and at a slightly faster pace.
- Adopt a staggered or wide stance.

## Exercise 11.6 • Woggle Jumps

### Purpose

This is a variation of the Tuck Jump. It is another high-intensity exercise that should be used specifically in the main workout. It can be combined with other exercises of moderate intensity to improve cardiovascular fitness.

### Starting position and instructions

Adopt a narrow straddled foot position. Bend the knees and push through the thigh muscles to create an upward motion through the water. The knees should move to the front of the chest and jump over the front of the woggle. The woggle can be used to push down through the water to assist the height of the movement achieved. Reverse the movement to jump backwards over the woggle.

### Coaching points

- Keep the knee joint unlocked.
- Ensure the heels go down when landing.
- Keep the elbows slightly bent throughout the movement.
- Keep the hips facing forwards.

### Progressions

- Start with a smaller tuck, just touching the knees to the woggle.
- Start at a slower pace and progressively increase the speed.
- Push the woggle down more forcefully through the water to increase the height of the jump and increase the overall intensity of the movement.

| Exercise 11.6 | Woggle Jumps |
| --- | --- |

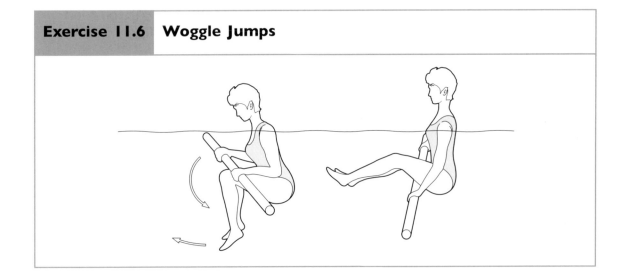

| Exercise 11.7 | Jump Twists with Water Bells |
| --- | --- |

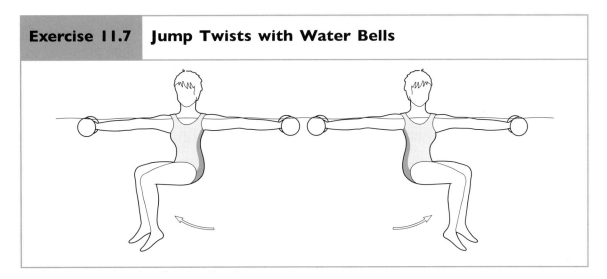

## Exercise 11.7 • Jump Twists with Water Bells

### Purpose

This exercise will strengthen the muscles at the front and side of the abdomen thoracic (rectus abdominus and obliques). It will also improve cardiovascular fitness.

### Starting position and instructions

Adopt a straddled foot position. Hold a water bell in each hand at the side of the body.

Jump and twist the body to the right and then back to the left. The water bells can be pulled through the water.

### Coaching points

- Keep the hips and knees facing forwards. Do not let the knee joint roll inwards.
- Keep the elbows unlocked.
- Make sure the lower back does not twist.
- Keep the arms under the water.

### Progressions

- Start with a small jump and progressively add height and power to the jump.
- Start slowly and progressively increase speed.

## Exercise 11.8 • Leg Kicks with Woggle

| Exercise 11.8 | Leg Kicks with Woggle |
| --- | --- |

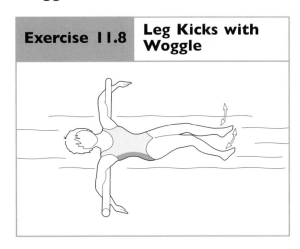

### Purpose

This exercise will work the muscles at the front and back of the hip and thigh (hip flexors, quadriceps, gluteals and hamstrings).

## Starting position and instructions

Lie on your back with the woggle underneath shoulders. Kick the legs as fast as you find comfortable.

## Coaching points

- Keep the abdominals pulled in.
- Ensure the lower back does not hollow.
- Keep the knee joints unlocked.
- Keep the hips square so that the lower spine does not twist.

## Progressions

- Start slowly and progressively kick faster and harder.
- Start with a smaller range of motion, then progress to working through a fuller range of motion.

# Exercise 11.9 • Pendulums Woggle Push

## Purpose

This exercise primarily assists with raising and maintaining the heart rate.

## Starting position and instructions

Adopt a narrow straddled foot position. Hop on to one leg, swinging the other leg to the side of the body and pushing the woggle across the front of the body, away from the swinging leg. Repeat by hopping on to the other leg and moving the arms in the opposite direction.

## Coaching points

- Keep the knee joint unlocked.
- Keep the elbows slightly bent.
- Keep the hips facing forwards.
- Ensure the heels go down.

## Progressions

- Start with a smaller hop and a lower swing of the leg.
- Progress by hopping slightly higher and swinging the leg out further.
- Rebound the body out of the water with each stride taken.
- Move at a slightly faster pace.
- Push the woggle more forcefully in the water.

| **Exercise 11.9** | **Pendulums Woggle Push** |
| --- | --- |

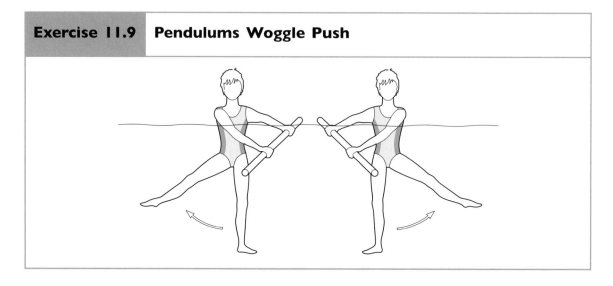

## Exercise 11.10 • Flip Over with Water Bells

### Purpose

To work the muscles at the front and side of the trunk (the rectus abdominus and obliques).

### Starting position and instructions

Lie face down and hold the water bells under the water in front of the body.

Contract the abdominal muscles and bend the knees towards the chest. Drag the legs through the water until you are lying on your back with the water bells by your hips and under the water. Contract the abdominals again and reverse the movement. Extend the legs once the buttocks are close to the surface of the water.

### Coaching points

- Ensure the lower back does not hollow as the legs return to the water surface.
- Keep the movement controlled.
- Keep the abdominals pulled in.
- Keep the head in line with the spine.

### Progressions:

- Start by performing the movement at half range (just front or just back).
- Combine the moves, but place the feet on the floor as a break between movements.
- Perform free floating, using sculling movements of the arms to maintain flotation.

**Exercise 11.10  Flip Over with Water Bells**

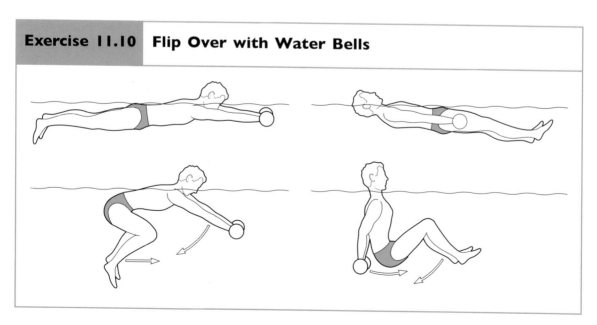

## Exercise 11.11 • Leg Scissors with Woggle

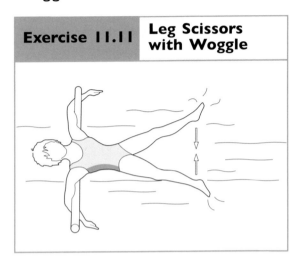

| Exercise 11.11 | Leg Scissors with Woggle |

## Exercise 11.12 • Breaststroke Legs with Woggle

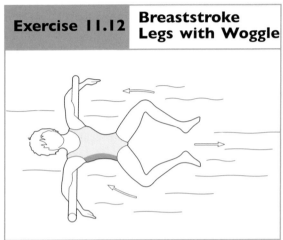

| Exercise 11.12 | Breaststroke Legs with Woggle |

### Purpose

This exercise will work the muscles on the inside and outside of the thigh and hip (the adductors and the abductors).

### Starting position and instructions

Lie on the back, holding the woggle under the shoulders. Allow the legs to float upwards to a level that is comfortable. The legs can stay low if that feels better. Take the legs apart as far as is comfortable, then draw them together and scissor one across the other.

### Coaching points

- Keep the knees unlocked.
- Keep the hips square.
- Maintain the natural curve of the lower back, but do not allow the back to hollow.

### Progressions

- Start slowly; progress by increasing the speed.
- Use ankle cuffs or fins to increase the surface area of the movement.

### Purpose

This exercise will work the buttock muscles (gluteals), and the muscles at the front and back of the thigh (quadriceps and hamstrings).

### Starting position and instructions

Lie on your back, holding the woggle under the shoulders. Allow the legs to float upwards to a level that is comfortable. The legs can stay low if it is easier. Bend the knees and draw the legs towards the armpits. Push the legs away to an extended position and repeat the movement.

### Coaching points

- Ensure the lower back does not hollow.
- Pull in the abdominals.
- Do not lock the knees.
- Keep the hips square.
- Keep the shoulders relaxed.

### Progressions

- Start at a slower pace and progress by working more quickly.
- Progress by adding ankle cuffs or water fins to the ankle to increase resistance.

## Exercise 11.13 • Bicep Curls with Water Bells

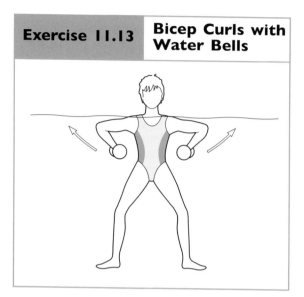

| Exercise 11.13 | **Bicep Curls with Water Bells** |
|---|---|

### Purpose

This exercise will work the muscles at the front of the arm (the biceps).

### Starting position and instructions

Adopt a staggered or straddled foot stance. Hold one water bell in each hand at the surface of the water. Drag the arms down through the water towards the armpits. Return the arms under control to the surface of the water.

### Coaching points

- Keep the elbows unlocked.
- Keep the hips facing forwards.
- Keep the abdominals pulled in.
- Keep the arms under water.

### Progressions

- Start by moving through a smaller range of motion, exerting less force against the water.
- Progress by moving through a larger range

of motion, moving at a slightly faster pace and exerting more force against the water.

## Exercise 11.14 • Woggle Ride and Jump

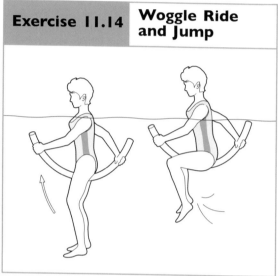

| Exercise 11.14 | **Woggle Ride and Jump** |
|---|---|

### Purpose

This exercise will elevate and maintain the heart rate. It can be either a moderate or high-intensity exercise depending on the height of the jump and whether turning is included.

### Starting position and instructions

Place the woggle in between the legs, holding one end of the woggle in each hand. Bend the knees and push through the thigh muscles to jump out of the water.

### Coaching points

- Keep the knee joint unlocked.
- Ensure the heels go down when landing.
- Keep the hips facing forwards.

## Progressions

- Start with a small jump and little rebound out of the water.
- Progress to a larger jump out of the water by exerting a greater force through the thighs and using the arms strongly.
- Travel forwards and backwards.

# Exercise 11.15 • Woggle Ride

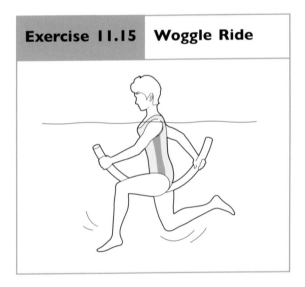

| Exercise 11.15 | Woggle Ride |
|---|---|

## Coaching points

- Keep the knee joint unlocked.
- Keep the hips facing forwards.
- Keep the abdominals pulled in.
- Ensure the shoulders are relaxed and down.

## Progressions

- Start with a smaller pedalling action of the legs and progress to a larger pedalling action.
- Exert a greater force through the thigh and use the arms if necessary.
- Travel the movement for a greater distance.

## Purpose

This exercise will maintain the heart rate. It is performed in a suspended state.

## Starting position and instructions

Place the woggle between the legs, raise the feet to sit on the woggle and suspend the body so that the legs are not in contact with the pool floor. Hold one end of the woggle in each hand. Use the hands to push the water down to assist flotation or travel if necessary. Use the legs to push the water down in a cycling action to assist flotation and create travel.

## Exercise 11.16 • Forward Punching with Delta Bells

### Purpose

This exercise will work the triceps muscles at the back of the upper arm and the pectoral muscles at the front of the chest when pushing forwards, and the biceps muscle at the front of the upper arm, the latissimus dorsi, the trapezius and the rhomboids (back muscles) when pulling backwards.

### Starting position and instructions

Adopt a staggered foot position. Hold the water bells with an overhand grip, and allow them to float at the water surface. Start punching the water bells alternately forwards and backwards through the water, fully extending the elbow.

### Coaching points

- Keep the abdominals pulled in.
- Keep the shoulders relaxed and down.
- Fully extend, but do not lock the elbows.
- Keep the knees unlocked.
- Keep the back straight.

### Progressions

- If using water bells or paddles, allow half of the equipment to stay out of the water, reducing the surface area.
- Work at a slower pace.
- Work through a smaller range of motion.
- Progress to working through a full range of motion and at a slightly faster pace.
- Punch down through the water to progress.
- Add Spotty Dog legs (*see* page 100) for additional cardiovascular work.

| Exercise 11.16 | Forward Punching with Delta Bells |
| --- | --- |

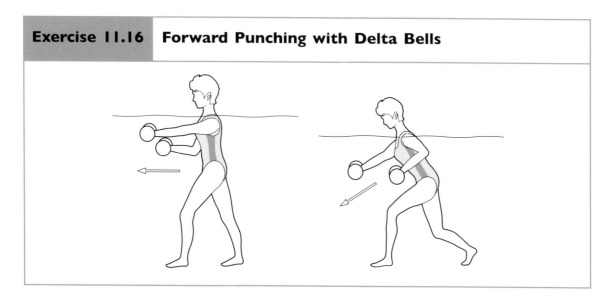

## Exercise 11.17 • Upper-cut Punching with Delta Bells

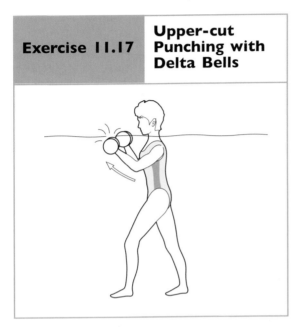

| Exercise 11.17 | **Upper-cut Punching with Delta Bells** |
|---|---|

### Coaching points

- Keep the abdominals pulled in.
- Keep the shoulders relaxed and down.
- Fully extend, but do not lock the elbows.
- Keep the knees unlocked.
- Keep the back straight.

### Progressions

- Work at a slower pace.
- Work through a smaller range of motion.
- Progress to working through a full range of motion and at a slightly faster pace.

### Purpose

This exercise will work the biceps muscles at the front of the upper arm, the pectoral muscles at the front of the chest and the deltoids (shoulders).

### Starting position and instructions

Adopt a staggered foot position. Hold the water bells in front of the body, elbows bent.

Start punching the water bells upwards, rolling them back and down through the water using a fast rolling action.

| Exercise 11.18 | **Lateral Press with Bells** |
| --- | --- |

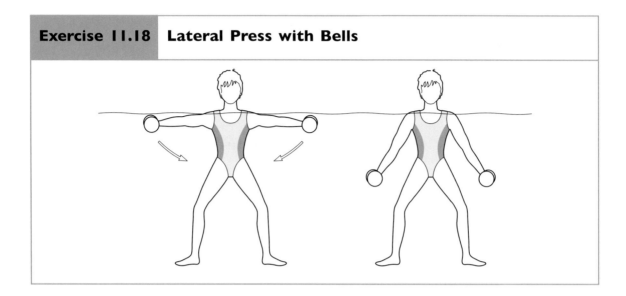

## Exercise 11.18 • Lateral Press with Bells

### Purpose

This exercise will work the pectoral muscles at the front of the chest when pushing forwards, and the latissimus dorsi and trapezius and rhomboids at the back when pushing to the back. The deltoids (shoulders) will also work.

### Starting position and instructions

Adopt a comfortable and stable foot position. Hold the water bells out to the sides of the body. Start pressing the equipment down through the water towards the thighs. Press alternately to the front and to the back.

### Coaching points

- Keep the abdominals pulled in.
- Keep the shoulders relaxed and down.
- Do not lock the elbows.
- Keep the knees unlocked.
- Keep the back straight.

### Progressions

- Work at a slower pace.
- Work through a smaller range of motion.
- Progress to working through a full range of motion and at a slightly faster pace.

## Deep-water training

### What is deep-water training?

Deep-water training occurs when the body is fully submerged in the water to neck depth and no contact is made with the pool floor throughout the programme. This requires the body to work in an open kinematic (without forces that bring out the motion) environment.

### What are the advantages and disadvantages of deep-water training?

There are a number of benefits from training in deep water. There are also some disadvantages. These are listed in table 11.1.

| Table 11.1 | The advantages and disadvantages of deep-water training |
|---|---|

| Advantages | Disadvantages |
|---|---|
| • Increased buoyancy and flotation.<br>• Impact forces are eliminated and joint stress is minimal.<br>• Improved range of motion due to weightlessness of the joints.<br>• Correct posture is required to keep the body in an upright, lengthened position.<br>• Excellent work for core trunk and pelvic stabilisers.<br>• Diaphragmatic breathing can be encouraged to work with additional hydrostatic pressure. This can promote cardiovascular conditioning.<br>• Increased resistance will enhance the effectiveness of the workout.<br>• Deep-water training covers the body totally. Individuals who are more body conscious will feel less exposed.<br>• Use of a buoyancy belt provides flotation and enables the body to move through a full range of motion.<br>• Buoyancy aids can be used to assist relaxation and stretching at the end of the session.<br>• Webbed gloves increase intensity of the workout. | • Some participants will feel unstable until they acclimatise to working in deeper water.<br>• Participants with weaker core muscles may find the programme tiring and will need rest breaks for these muscles.<br>• Hydrostatic pressure will increase, which will make breathing feel more difficult and may give the impression of a harder workout.<br>• Participants with respiratory problems may find it uncomfortable to work in deep water.<br>• Increased resistance may make the body feel heavier. Movements will need to be slower.<br>• Teachers will need to make movements slower and allow more time for transitions.<br>• Equipment is essential to maintain flotation and provide support to the body. |

## NEED TO KNOW

• Diaphragmatic breathing is the method of breathing encouraged during Pilates-based training. It consists of encouraging the breath to move deeper into the lungs – the side and back of the lower ribcage expand out sideways and backwards during inhalation.

To practise this technique:
• Place the hands around the lower ribcage (thumbs around the back of the ribs).
• As you breathe in, the ribcage should move slightly and press into the hands and thumbs.
• As you breathe out, the ribcage will relax.

## What type of exercise can be used in a deep-water session?

The exercises that can be used in a deep-water session are:
* Jogging
* Ski Strides
* Jumping Jacks
* Kicking
* Cycling
* Rocking Horse
* Farmer Giles

### Fig. 11.9   Jogging

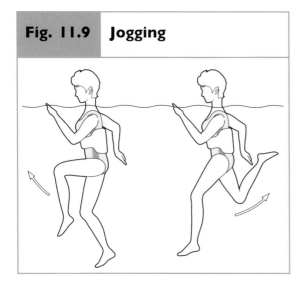

**Variations:** travel, knees high, heels to buttocks, vertical, horizontal, raise one arm out of water, raise both arms out of water.

### Fig. 11.10   Ski Strides

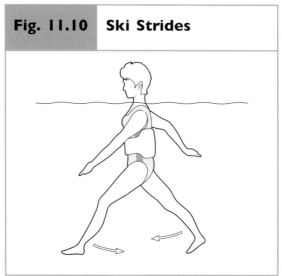

**Variations:** neutral, rebound, combine with Jumping Jacks.

### Fig. 11.11   Jumping Jacks

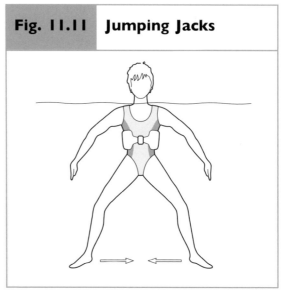

**Variations:** neutral, rebound, combine with Ski Strides, add to end of travel movement.

| Fig. 11.12 | Kicking |
| --- | --- |

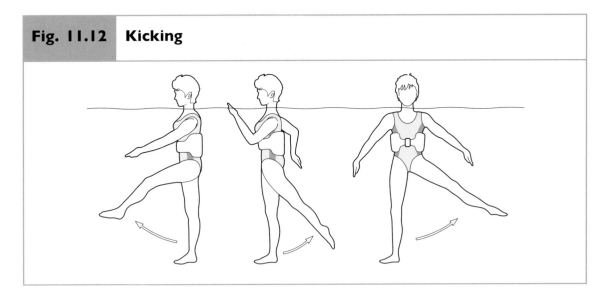

**Variations:** kick forwards, kick sideways, kick backwards, add arm lines and travel, turn, increase lever, perform vertical or seated kicks.

| Fig. 11.13 | Cycling |
| --- | --- |

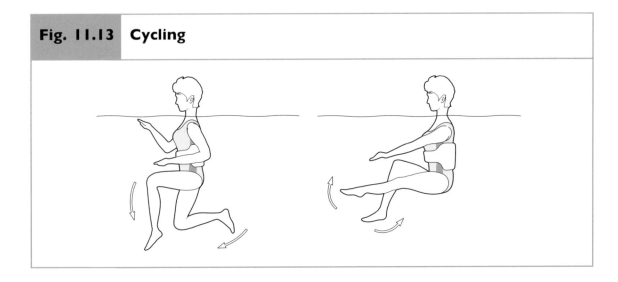

**Variations:** vertical cycling, horizontal cycling.

In addition, many of the exercises listed using other equipment can be adapted to work in deeper water.

## Main teaching points for a deep-water session

- Maintain upright posture.
- Keep the knees unlocked.
- Keep the pelvis neutral.
- Engage abdominals – creating a zipping up and hollowing feeling.
- Ensure the shoulders are relaxed and down.
- Keep the neck lengthened.
- Ensure your arm movements are controlled.
- Keep the elbows unlocked.

## How can these movements be developed?

1 The working position can be adapted to include:
   - horizontal lying
   - vertical standing neutral
   - vertical standing propulsive
   - seated position.
2 The speed of the move can be varied.
3 Travel and direction changes can be added.
4 Movements that work through different planes can be combined, e.g Jumping Jacks and Ski Strides.
5 Levers can be made longer.
6 The arm lines can be varied and used either:
   - submerged under the water
   - out of the water (not too frequently as this may elevate blood pressure)
   - at the water surface.

| Fig. 11.14 | **Rocking Horse** |
|---|---|

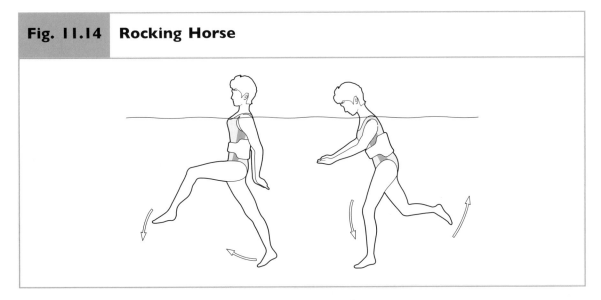

**Variations:** add travel, extend levers, neutral, rebound.

| **Fig. 11.15** | **Farmer Giles** |

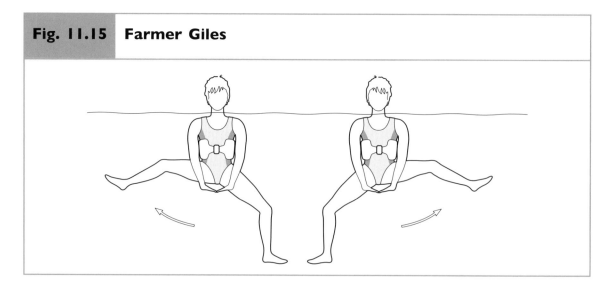

**Variations:** extend levers, neutral, rebound, raise one arm out of the water, raise both arms out of the water.

## SHORT ANSWER REVISION QUESTIONS

1. State **THREE** advantages of using equipment in a water-based session.

2. State **THREE** disadvantages of using equipment in a water-based session.

3. Describe **TWO** ways of using:
   (a) woggles
   (b) water bells
   (c) frisbees
   (d) floats
   (e) mitts
   (f) water vests or buoyancy belts
   (g) ankle cuffs.

4. State **THREE** advantages of deep-water training.

5. State **THREE** disadvantages of deep-water training.

6. Describe **FOUR** ways movements will need to be adapted for deep water.

# DESIGNING A CIRCUIT TRAINING PROGRAMME

## OBJECTIVES

By the end of this chapter the reader will be able to:

- State some of the benefits of circuit training in a water-based session
- Recognise how to structure a circuit session in water
- Identify a range of circuit designs that can be used within a water-based exercise session
- Recognise different methods of controlling a circuit
- Describe how to adapt the timing, intensity and structure of a circuit session in water to accommodate different needs and requirements.

## Why use a circuit training format?

Circuit training can provide an effective alternative to the traditional structure of a water-based exercise programme. Circuit training offers great flexibility and versatility and enables the potential for a variety of cardiovascular and muscular strength and endurance training approaches to be integrated in the session. The timing of the work/rest ratios can be structured to bring about an interval training approach. Specific stations can be designed to use some of the resistance training approaches. Circuits also enable a variety of equipment to be used within the session. They can be designed to train all the components of fitness, and will add variety to the programme for regular water exercisers. It may also attract interest from new participants.

## How should a circuit training programme be structured?

The session should be preceded by an appropriate warm-up and concluded with an appropriate warm-down. The main workout should comprise a range of exercises designed in a circuit training format. An outline of the necessary session structure is given in table 12.1.

## What exercises are appropriate for use in the circuit?

If the aim of the circuit is purely to improve cardiovascular fitness, all of the exercises illustrated at the end of Chapters 8 and 9 will be appropriate. If the aim of the circuit is to improve muscular strength and endurance, the exercises illustrated at the end of Chapter 10

| Table 12.1 | The structure of a circuit training session |
| --- | --- |

**Warm-up**
- Mobility and pulse-raising activities
- Preparatory stretches
- Re-warm (increasing intensity to the level of the circuit)

**Main workout – circuit training component (three approaches)**
1. Specific toning exercises targeting all major muscle groups to achieve a balanced whole body approach and improve muscular strength and endurance, or . . .
2. A range of exercises to improve cardiovascular fitness, or . . .
3. A combination of both types of exercises to improve each component of fitness

**Cool-down**
- Cooling down exercises (lowering intensity from the level of the circuit)
- Post-workout stretches
- Relaxation activities (optional)
- Re-mobilise.

**Note:** the intensity and selection of exercises included in the re-warmer and cool-down will need to correspond to the intensity of the main workout. If the intensity of the main workout is high and includes a number of energetic cardiovascular movements, then the intensity of these components will need to be built up and built down from this higher level of intensity respectively. Guidelines for building and lowering the intensity to a higher level are discussed in Chapter 6 and Chapter 8.

will be appropriate. If a combined cardiovascular fitness and muscular strength and endurance workout is to be achieved, then the exercises in all of the aforementioned chapters are appropriate.

When using a combined approach, it is wise to alternate muscular strength and endurance exercises with cardiovascular exercises. This should ensure that the intensity of activities is maintained for an appropriate frequency to make cardiovascular fitness improvements. This approach is advisable because some of the muscular strength and endurance activities illustrated are less demanding on the cardiovascular system. They may lower the intensity too much if performed consecutively in the same circuit.

An alternative approach is to perform two specific circuits, the first circuit consisting of cardiovascular exercises, and the second consisting of muscular strength and endurance exercises. If two main circuits are used then the intensity of the cardiovascular circuit will need to be reduced slightly before going on to the muscular strength and endurance circuit. An appropriate session structure to follow for this approach is outlined in table 8.1 on page 125.

## How can the circuit be controlled?

If performing a circuit of water-based exercises as part of our own training, we need quite simply to plan the activities and then head for the water. However, instructors who are dealing with groups of participants will need to plan carefully to ensure adequate control is achieved. Participants will need to be introduced to the stations, otherwise they may be unsure of how to perform the exercises correctly. Some instructors introduce stations after the re-warmer but this approach often lowers the intensity, unless participants are kept sufficiently active while the exercises are being demonstrated and explained. A more appropriate method of introducing the exercise stations is to perform each exercise at a lower intensity throughout the warm-up component. This will assist with a progressive rise in intensity, maintain interest, and improve the continuity of the session.

Unfortunately, participants may still forget stations when the main circuit is in operation. The use of printed circuit training cards to illustrate the exercise to be performed at each station, can act as a reminder. The diagrams need to be large, clear, and visible, and the cards will need to be laminated for use on the poolside. It is also useful if key coaching points are listed as safety reminders.

The use of assistant instructors and spotters may also assist with effective control. However, they will need to be instructed carefully about their role and responsibilities. In reality, assistants are not frequently accessible. Therefore, if dealing with inexperienced groups without assistance, it is often easier to reduce the number of stations being performed around the pool at the same time. Figs 12.3, 12.4 and 12.5 on page 200 illustrate appropriate approaches for dealing with less experienced groups.

## What circuit formats are available?

There are a number of ways a group can be organised to perform the main circuit training component. The format selected should be appropriate to the number of stations and participants. If dealing with smaller groups it is unwise to have a large number of stations with only one person exercising on each. It is advisable to encourage a group of people to perform at each station to assist with group motivation and observation. Five different formats are illustrated in Figs 12.1 to 12.5. Some of the advantages and disadvantages for using each of the different formats are also identified.

| **Figure 12.1 Square circuit – traditional** | | | |
|---|---|---|---|
| 1 XXXX | 2 XXXX | 3 XXXX | 4 XXXX |
| XXXX 5 | XXXX 6 | XXXX 7 | XXXX 8 |

### Advantages

- Can use all water depths.
- Can position exercises at an appropriate water depth.
- Can have a large number of stations.
- Variety of stations should maintain interest.

### Disadvantages

- Harder for the instructor to move around and observe.
- Water depth may not be appropriate for all.

**Figure 12.2 Lined circuit**

| 1 | 2 | 3 | 4 | 5 | 6 | 7 | 8 |
|---|---|---|---|---|---|---|---|
| X | X | X | X | X | X | X | X |
| X | X | X | X | X | X | X | X |
| X | X | X | X | X | X | X | X |
| X | X | X | X | X | X | X | X |
| X | X | X | X | X | X | X | X |
| X | X | X | X | X | X | X | X |
| X | X | X | X | X | X | X | X |

## Advantages

- Works well for cardiovascular circuits.
- Relatively easy to move around and observe.
- Can position stations in the appropriate water depths.

## Disadvantages

- Works less effectively for muscular strength and endurance circuits because poolside space is limited.
- Difficult, if not impossible, to organise and use equipment for this approach.
- Water depth selected may not be appropriate for all individuals when changing lines.

**Figure 12.3 Corners circuit**

| 1 | 2 |
|---|---|
| XXXX | XXXX |
| XXXX | XXXX |
| XXXX | XXXX |
| | |
| | |
| XXXX | XXXX |
| XXXX | XXXX |
| XXXX | XXXX |
| 3 | 4 |

## Advantages

- Easier to manage due to fewer stations.
- Ideal for smaller groups.
- Ideal for beginners: fewer exercises to remember and repetition could improve performance.
- Very small groups can perform at one station and the instructor can move around with them to assist performance.

## Disadvantages

- May need a spotter to assist with observation if pool is large.
- May become too repetitious or boring if the same stations are repeated for a number of circuits.

**Figure 12.4 Half split circuit**

| 1 | 2 |
|---|---|
| XXXXXXXXX | XXXXXXXXX |
| XXXXXXXXX | XXXXXXXXX |
| XXXXXXXXX | XXXXXXXXX |
| XXXXXXXXX | XXXXXXXXX |
| XXXXXXXXX | XXXXXXXXX |
| XXXXXXXXX | XXXXXXXXX |
| XXXXXXXXX | XXXXXXXXX |
| XXXXXXXXX | XXXXXXXXX |

## Advantages

- Easier to manage: only two exercises being performed at the same time.
- Can perform deep and shallow exercises consecutively (need a spotter and lifeguard for deep-water activities).
- Easy to lead and instruct beginners: fewer exercises to explain.

## Disadvantages

- May need a spotter to observe one half of group if pool is large.
- Transition times to each side of the pool can be long, especially if equipment is used.

| Figure 12.5 Scattered – command led circuit |
|---|
| X    X    X    X<br>X    X    X    X    X<br>X    X    X    X<br>X    X    X    X    X<br>X    X    X    X<br>X    X    X    X    X<br>X    X    X    X |

## Advantages

- All participants perform the same activity at the same time.
- Only commands for one exercise need to be given at one time.
- No circuit cards are needed: participants follow instructor's commands.
- Can control large groups more easily.
- Can adapt for mixed ability groups and beginners more easily.
- Can allow participants to select and vary the depth of water they work in to suit the activity.

## Disadvantages

- Space in appropriate water depth may be limited.
- Will need to offer alternative ways of performing activities if water is too shallow or deep for selected exercise.

# How can work time at each station be controlled?

The time spent working on a specific station or exercise can be dictated by either timing each exercise, or by specifying the number of repetitions to be performed. Both will require the establishment of an appropriate work time at each station and an appropriate rest time between stations. The work/rest ratio will need to be appropriate for the target group. Guidelines for appropriate work/rest ratios are provided in table 12.2 on page 202.

## The time-controlled circuit

There are two approaches to timing a circuit. The first approach is to measure the work and rest time using a stopwatch. A disadvantage of this approach is that more attention may be paid to watching the clock rather than participants. However, it does allow for the same time to be spent on each station. When proficient, it is possible to estimate the time rather than 'clock watch'.

Alternatively, a specific station can control the timing. For example, if Water Wading is used as a station, a set number of widths can be waded before moving on to the next station. A disadvantage of using this approach is that different participants may perform at different speeds. If some take longer, then the overall work time on each station will vary slightly.

## The repetition-controlled circuit

There are two approaches to controlling the repetitions performed. Either the instructor can dictate a set repetition range (e.g. 15 repetitions of each exercise), or they can allow participants to select from between two and four different repetition ranges (e.g. choose to perform either 8, 12, 16 or 20 repetitions of each exercise).

If the instructor sets only one number of repetitions, the quantity they suggest may not be appropriate for different abilities. However, this need not be a problem. Alternative intensities can be offered, and participants can be advised to select the alternative they can perform for the prescribed repetitions. However, some may perform at different speeds and may finish the exercise before others. This is equally a problem if a selection of repetition ranges are offered.

If participants select their different repetition ranges, some will finish before others. They will therefore be inactive while they wait for others to finish, and queues may develop at specific stations. The best way to avoid queues is to have a control exercise in the middle of the pool. Participants should perform the exercise while they wait for the rest of the group to complete their exercise. When the whole group are in the middle of the pool, everyone can move on to their next station.

## How can a circuit training session be adapted for different fitness levels?

The intensity of the individual stations can be adapted to suit different requirements by varying:
• the speed of the exercise
• the length of levers moved
• the range of motion
• the position (i.e. Side Leg Raises will be easier than Scissor Legs)
• the force exerted against the water
• the equipment
• the surface area of levers.

The intensity of the whole circuit training programme can be adapted to accommodate different needs by altering:
• the number of stations

• the intensity of the exercises at each station
• the time working at each station
• the rest time between each station
• the number of times the circuit is performed
• the rest time between each circuit
• the approach to circuit – giant sets or tri set circuit will be harder than other approaches (see example formats at end of the chapter).

More specific guidelines for adapting the intensity and duration of the circuit to accommodate different groups are given in table 12.2.

**Note:** Detailed progressions are provided for all the exercises illustrated in Chapters 8, 9 and 10.

| Table 12.2 | Adapting the intensity and duration of the circuit for different groups | | |
|---|---|---|---|
| Method of screening | Less fit and specialist groups | Intermediate fitness level and general groups | Advanced fitness level and sport – specific groups |
| Overall duration of circuit (including warm-up and cool-down) | 30–45 minutes | 45–60 minutes | 60 minutes |
| Overall intensity of circuit stations | Low | Moderate-high | Higher |
| Work time on station Note: if muscular strength is a goal then the time will need to be shorter and the intensity higher | Shorter | Moderate | Longer |
| Rest time between stations Note: cardiovascular circuits will need an active rest. Performing a lower intensity activity between stations should be sufficient | Longer rest time – performing lower intensity activity to allow sufficient recovery | Moderate rests – performing a moderately intense activity to allow recovery from higher intensity activities | Shorter rest time needed between more intense activities. Rest periods can be more active: aim for continuous movement around circuit |
| Approach Note: this may vary to accommodate the fitness goals of the individual/ group being trained | Timed or reps. Command format is easier to manage | Timed or reps | Timed or reps to tailor programme to meet specific needs |
| Number of stations Note: this may vary depending on the number of participants | Low (4–8) | Moderate (8–12) | Higher (10–20) depending on number of participants |

| Table 12.2 | Adapting the intensity and duration of the circuit for different groups (cont.) | | |
|---|---|---|---|
| Method of screening | Less fit and specialist groups | Intermediate fitness level and general groups | Advanced fitness level and sport – specific groups |
| Number of circuits Note: this may vary depending on the number of stations used | Low (1–2) | Moderate (1–3) | Higher (1–4) |
| Appropriate exercises All the exercises are illustrated at the end of Chapters 8, 9 and 10 | Compound (working a number of muscles to reduce the number of exercises) | Compound and isolation exercises using equipment | Compound and isolation exercises using equipment |

Note: Compound exercises can be more intense than some isolation exercises. Therefore, the intensity may need to be lowered for less fit exercisers and specialist groups.

## Example: CV lined circuit

**Work time** – vary to suit fitness level.
**Rest** – none. Move directly to next station or have group control exercise in centre of pool.
**Warm up before circuit and cool down after circuit.**

Station Number:
1. Jump Jacks
2. Sploosh and Turn
3. Shuttle Runs
4. Tuck Jumps
5. Side Squats
6. Ballet Jumps
7. Spotty Dogs
8. Flick Kicks
9. Woggle Jumps
10. Sploosh – no turns.

## Example: Easy CV/MSE circuit – square layout

**Work time** – vary to suit fitness level.
**Rest time** – jog to next station.
**Warm up before circuit and cool down after circuit.**

Station Number:
1. Jump Jacks
2. Sweep Through
3. Shuttle Runs
4. Twisters
5. Tuck Jumps
6. Press-ups
7. Ballet Jumps
8. Bicep Curl with water bells.

| Table 12.3 | Example: MSE/CV giant set circuit with active CV recovery | | |
|---|---|---|---|
| Station 1<br>Trunk | Mermaids | Twisters | Sweep Throughs |
| Station 2<br>Upper | Bear Hugs | Chest Press with<br>water bells | Water Punches |
| Station 3<br>Lower body<br>and CV | Scissor Legs | Jump Jacks | Pendulum |
| Station 4<br>CV | Sploosh | Tuck Jumps | Farmer Giles |
| Station 5<br>Arms | Elbow Curl | Press-ups out of pool | Bicep Curl with<br>water bells |

## Example: MSE/CV giant set circuit with active CV recovery

**Warm up before circuit and cool down after circuit**

**Work time per exercise:** 30 seconds – complete all exercises for one station before moving to next station (total 1½ minutes).

**Active rest:** Any CV or step-based move for 1½ minutes.

**Total time:** 15 minutes for one circuit or 30 minutes for two circuits. NB: different exercises can be used for second circuit.

NB: Work time can be decreased or increased to adapt for different levels. Active CV rest phase can be increased or decreased. Exercises can be varied and more equipment can be used.

## Example: Tri-circuit (CV and MSE focus)

**Warm up before circuit and cool down after circuit**

**Work time per exercise:** 1 minute (total 3 minutes). Perform each exercise per station before moving on to next station.

**Active rest:** Jog in place, or run around pool or in centre of pool for 1 minute.

**Total time:** 32 minutes for one circuit.

NB: Work time can be decreased or increased to adapt for different levels. Active rest can be increased for longer recovery. Exercises can be varied and more equipment can be used.

| Table 12.4 | Example: Tri-circuit (CV and MSE focus) | | |
|---|---|---|---|
| Station number | CV exercise | MSE equipment exercise | MSE exercise – no equipment |
| 1 | Sploosh | Chest Press with water bells | Mermaids |
| 2 | Tuck Jumps | Bicep Curls with water bells | Twisters |
| 3 | Jump Jacks | Rotator Cuff with woggles | Sweep Throughs |
| 4 | Farmer Giles | Press-ups out of pool | Scissor Legs |
| 5 | Pendulums | Flip Over with water bell | Mermaids |
| 6 | Ballet Jumps | Forward Punches with water bells | Twisters |
| 7 | Shuttle Runs | Upper Cuts with water bells | Sweep Throughs |
| 8 | Pike Jumps | Leg Kicks with woggles | Scissor Legs |

# SHORT ANSWER REVISION QUESTIONS

1. State **TWO** benefits of using a circuit approach in a water-based session.
2. Name **TWO** ways a circuit can be designed (stations arranged).
3. State **TWO** ways the work and rest time can be controlled.
4. Describe how the intensity, duration and content of a circuit exercise in water session can be adapted to accommodate different fitness levels.

# SPECIALIST PROGRAMMES

# PART FOUR

4

# AQUATIC TRAINING FOR SPORTSPEOPLE

13

## OBJECTIVES

By the end of this chapter the reader will be able to:

- Recognise some of the benefits of training in water for sportspeople
- Review the properties of water and how they may assist training with sportspeople
- Recognise the use of water-based exercises during different training seasons
- Identify a range of exercises that can be included for specific sporting needs.

Sportspeople are always at risk of overtraining and building up the intensity of their programmes too quickly. The occurrence of repetitive strain and overuse injuries are common. Training or cross training in water can improve and maintain physical fitness and assist with the development of specific skills. The main advantage of exercising in water is that the body is supported, and the risk of injury to the athlete is lower.

This chapter explores the benefits of exercising in water specifically for the sportsperson. It also outlines an appropriate session structure, and provides guidelines for designing a sport-specific programme.

## What are the benefits of water-based training for the sportsperson?

**Buoyancy** supports the bodyweight and decreases the impact and stress placed on joints.

Movements such as running, jumping, turning, and explosive power movements, are cushioned when performed in water. There is less risk of injury to the joints and muscles. Therefore, specific skill-related activities can be performed and repeated for much longer in water with far less potential risk of repetitive strain.

Water also provides **resistance** to the body's movements from all directions. The harder you pull, push or kick the water, the greater will be the resistance to your movement. This resistance provides many benefits for the sportsperson. There is less likelihood of reaching the end of the range of motion too quickly, so activities that replicate those performed in the specific sporting activity can be undertaken without the risk of damage to the tissues that surround the joints. Swinging a cricket bat or tennis racket through the water will be less stressful than when performed on land, but the muscles will be forced to work harder to overcome the water resistance. This can enhance performance in the specific sporting activity but without overstraining the muscles or joints.

The intensity of the activities can be built up progressively by using equipment that further increases the resistance provided to movement. Strapping water mitts to the tennis racket will increase the surface area and drag. Strapping other buoyancy devices to a cricket bat will increase flotation and surface area. Both will intensify the work necessary for the muscles to overcome the added resistance to movement, and will optimise the training benefits received.

# Why would a sportsperson exercise in water?

The sportsperson may turn to water-based training for a number of reasons:
- Pre-season training or cross training
- Main season cross training
- Post-season training or cross training
- Injury rehabilitation.

## Pre-season

The primary aim of pre-season training is to develop a base level of fitness in all components of physical fitness. These include muscular strength, muscular endurance, cardiovascular fitness, and flexibility. Once a base level of fitness is achieved, the sportsperson can then work towards developing the specific skills that will enhance their performance in their chosen sporting event. These will vary depending on the sporting activity, but may include one or more of the following: power, speed, balance, agility, co-ordination, etc. (Guidelines for improving fitness in each of these components are given in Chapter 2.) Water is a more supportive medium for training to improve fitness and develop skills. It will provide a release to the stress placed on the body from other pre-season land-based activities.

## Main season

During main season training, the sportsperson will need to develop and enhance their sport-specific skills further. Cross training in water will lessen the risk of injury that may be higher when training to improve these skills on land. Specific skill-related activities can be performed longer in water because the body is supported by buoyancy. Potentially cross training in water can assist with the fine tuning of specific skills and movements, without causing strain to the muscles or joints.

## Post-season

The primary aim of post-season training is to provide an active recovery period for the body. The body will need time to recuperate and recover from the stresses placed on it from competitive activity. The programme of activities provided at this stage should be sufficient to maintain a reasonable level of physical fitness, but they should be less demanding. A greater emphasis can be placed on mobility and stretching activities. Exercising in water can maintain fitness and can enhance mobility and stretching activities. The additional benefit of exercising in water during post-season training is that the pressure of the water against the body will create a massaging effect. This will assist the relaxation of the body and help to reduce physical and mental tension.

## Injury rehabilitation

Injury can leave the sportsperson feeling frustrated. They will be desperate to get back to their training regime and restore their fitness level. Water is supportive to the body, so it is possible for them to continue training in water when recovering from an injury. Fitness can be developed, and skills enhanced, without placing the injured joint or muscle under so much stress.

The use of a buoyancy belt, even for shallower water workouts, will provide further support to the body and reduce the risk of causing further trauma. In addition, the pressure of the water may help to reduce the swelling and reduce the pain at the injured site. It is advisable that specific injury rehabilitation programmes are developed with the guidance of a physiotherapist.

# How should the sport-specific training session be structured?

Sport-specific training should follow the same session structure as any other session. The session should be preceded by an adequate period of warming up, and concluded with an adequate period of warming down. The design of the main session will be dependent on the athlete's reasons for participating. It is wise to include activities to improve all components of physical fitness. However, specific attention may need to be given to:

- replicating the activities performed maximally throughout the sport
- counter-balancing the strength of the opposing muscles to those used maximally throughout the activity
- developing flexibility in muscles that are required to lengthen quickly when their opposing muscle is contracted quite forcefully. (For example, to kick a ball the quadriceps contract forcefully. Their opposing muscle group, the hamstrings, needs to be sufficiently flexible to relax and lengthen. If the hamstrings are not flexible, there is a greater risk of the muscle tearing.)

An appropriate session structure is outlined in table 13.1.

| Table 13.1 | Structuring a sport-specific training session |
| --- | --- |

**Warm-up**
- Mobility and pulse-raising: target joints used through the main workout.
- Preparatory stretches: include extra static or range of motion stretches for muscles that will need to move through an extended range of motion during the main workout.
- Re-warm specific to the main activity.

**Main workout**
- Include activities to train cardiovascular fitness.
- Include activities to replicate activities of the specific sport (skill, power, etc.).
- Include activities to strengthen opposing muscle groups to counter-balance and compensate for overuse in sporting activities.

**Cool-down**
- Cool-down activities to lower heart rate should be specific to the main activity.
- Stretch all muscles worked.
- Develop less flexible muscles if pool temperature allows.

**Note:** a circuit training session works well for training sportspeople.

# How can an effective sport-specific training programme be developed?

To design an effective sport-specific training session, it is necessary to identify the main movement activities used in the sport. Identifying how the joints move and how the muscles contract will assist with the selection of appropriate activities. Observing a video recording of a sporting activity will allow the instructor to analyse and break down the movements more specifically. Once the main activities have been identified, it is necessary to identify ways of replicating these movements in water. Table 13.2 provides a very basic breakdown of two of the activities used when playing soccer.

Even this basic analysis of the movements provides evidence that the quadriceps muscles receive a greater amount of work than their antagonist, the hamstrings. The following activities should therefore be considered:

- Strengthening work for the quadriceps and hip flexors as the main prime movers.
- Counter-balancing strengthening work for the hamstrings.
- Flexibility work for the hamstrings and gluteals to ensure these muscles have sufficient range of motion to lengthen when their opposing muscles contract so forcefully.
- Flexibility work for all muscles that are contracting strongly throughout the activity, i.e. quadriceps, gastrocnemius, soleus, erector spinae, to maintain flexibility.
- Improvement of cardiovascular fitness.
- Improvement of anaerobic fitness through explosive bursts.

| **Table 13.2** | **Breakdown of the joint actions and muscles working for two of the main activities in soccer** | | |
|---|---|---|---|
| Movement | Joint action | Prime mover (muscle that contracts to bring about the movement) | Antagonist (muscle that lengthens when prime mover contracts) |
| Kicking | Hip flexion | Hip flexor; quadriceps | Gluteals, hamstrings |
| Kicking | Knee extension | Quadriceps | Hamstring |
| Running | Hip flexion | Hip flexor; quadriceps | Gluteals, hamstrings |
| Running | Hip extension | Gluteals, hamstrings | Hip flexor; quadriceps |
| Running | Ankle dorsi flexion | Tibialis anterior | Gastrocnemius Soleus |
| Running | Ankle plantar flexion | Gastrocnemius soleus | Tibialis anterior |
| Running | Knee extension | Quadriceps | Hamstrings |

# Suggested activities for the main workouts of four different sport-specific programmes

## Soccer – main workout

Ten circuit stations: perform the complete circuit twice through.

1 Running widths of the pool, in navel to chest depth water, travelling forwards for one width and backwards for one width. (Repeat three times, and use to time and control the circuit.)
2 Deep-water jog and sprint with buoyancy belt: power legs up.
3 Pool Press-ups for upper body balance (page 169).
4 Tuck Jumps – chest depth (page 135).
5 Combined Sweep Through and Float and Pull for abdominals (pages 163–64).
6 Flick Kicks travelling back with rebound (page 103).
7 Jog Heels to Bottom – fast and slow (page 99).
8 Headers with partner. Partner A throws the ball and partner B jumps to head the ball back to A. Repeat six times and then change over so that B throws the ball and A heads the ball.
9 Tag with partner. A runs anywhere in pool, B tags A. On second circuit, B is tagged by A.
10 Flip Flaps (page 168).

### Other ideas for soccer

1 Team game tag. One team member chases rest of team. As each team member is tagged they join original team member in chase to tag rest of team.
2 Group headers (static or on the move).

## Boxing – main workout

Ten circuit stations: perform circuit twice through.

1 Water Pushes with water bells (page 104).
2 Shadow box: punch and block through air (waist depth).
3 Float and Pull with buoyancy belt and water bell(s) between knees (page 164).
4 Jumping Jacks (page 137).
5 Shadow box and punch through water (chest depth).
6 Spotty Dogs (page 100).
7 Tuck Jumps (page 135).
8 Deep water shadow box with buoyancy belt and punch through water.
9 Pool Press-ups (page 169).
10 Bear Hugs (page 170).

### Flexibility focus for boxing

Pectorals, triceps, latissimus dorsi, trapezius, hamstrings, gastrocnemius, hip flexor, adductors.

## Basketball – main workout

Ten circuit stations: perform the complete circuit twice through.

1 Leap Frogs (page 134).
2 Ski Jumps over step (page 147).
3 Running widths of the pool, in navel to chest depth water, travelling forwards for one width and backwards for one width. (Repeat three times and use to time and control the circuit.)
4 Jump, throw and catch with partner.
5 Tag with partner. Partner A runs anywhere in pool, partner B tags A. On second circuit, B is tagged by A.
6 Pool Press-ups (page 169).
7 Sploosh (page 138).
8 Mermaids (page 161).
9 Treading Water (page 139).
10 Power Lunges using step and ball (push ball through water) (page 152).

### Other ideas for basketball

1 Practise shots in water to decrease impact (can wear buoyancy belt as further cushion).

2 Team game tag.

3 Team basketball in water. Replace ball bounce and pass with push ball down through water and pass.

### Flexibility focus for basketball

Latissimus dorsi, obliques, pectorals, trapezius, triceps, hamstrings, hip flexor, quadriceps, adductors.

## Rugby – main workout

Ten circuit stations: perform the complete circuit twice through.

1 Running widths of the pool, in navel to chest depth water, travelling forwards for one width and backwards for one width with rugby ball. (Repeat three times and use to time and control the circuit.)

2 Deep water jog and sprint with buoyancy belt and rugby ball.

3 Bear Hugs (page 170).

4 Spotty Dogs (page 100).

5 Float and Pull with buoyancy belt and water bell(s) between knees (page 164).

6 Tag with partner. Partner A runs anywhere in pool, partner B tags A. On second circuit, B is tagged by A.

7 Tuck Jumps (page 135).

8 Tag and tackle with partner. Partner A runs with ball, partner B chases with aim of gaining possession of ball. When B has possession, A takes chase.

9 Jumping Jacks (page 137).

10 Jog Heels to Bottom – fast and slow (page 99).

### Other ideas for rugby

1 Scrum in water.

2 Team game. Bulldog: half of team line up to form a barrier across the pool. Rest of team line up at one end of the pool and run with the ball, aiming to break through the team barrier and place the ball on the pool wall at the other side.

### Flexibility focus for rugby

Hamstrings, gastrocnemius, quadriceps, adductors, hip flexor, pectorals, latissimus dorsi, and obliques.

## Running and walking – main workout

Runners and walkers can be trained effectively in water. The following elements can be varied to alter the effect of the training:

- Water depth: waist or chest deep. (Note: there will be greater stress placed on the body if running in waist depth water.)
- Equipment: with or without buoyancy belt, with or without water bells.
- Direction: static, travelling forwards and backwards, travelling in all directions.
- Speed: slow, moderate, fast sprint.
- Stride length: small, normal, large.
- Mode: rebounding, neutral or suspended. (Different modes are described in Chapter 8.)

### Flexibility focus for running and walking

Hamstrings, adductors, hip flexors, gastrocnemius, tibialis anterior, quadriceps.

## Dancing – main workout

1 Perform movement sequences and choreography patterns in water. The water provides increased resistance to movements, so the muscles will need to work harder to overcome the resistance.

2 Perform specific leaping and jumping movements for a longer duration. Water will provide support and reduce the stress placed on the body. It will also assist the development of correct technique: if technique is not

accurate, balance will be lost when re-entering the water.

3 Perform barre work at poolside: water will assist the duration for which the positions can be held. A greater range of motion may also be achieved.

## SHORT ANSWER REVISION QUESTIONS

1. State **TWO** benefits of exercising in water with sportspeople.
2. State **TWO** disadvantages of exercising in water with sportspeople.
3. Describe the effects of water and how they may affect water-based training with sportspeople.
4. Describe how water-based exercise can be used during different training seasons.
5. List some of the key considerations for session structure and content when working with sportspeople.

# AQUATIC TRAINING WITH OLDER ADULTS

14

## OBJECTIVES

By the end of this session the reader will be able to:

- Identify some of the physiological changes associated with the ageing process
- Recognise some appropriate considerations for adapting the water-based session to work with apparently healthy older adults
- Realise the need for further training to work effectively and safely with older adults, in particular those with other specialist requirements (exercise referral).

Physical activity is beneficial no matter what age we start exercising. The rate at which we progress, however, will be slightly slower when we are older.

This chapter discusses the effects of ageing on the body, the benefits of exercising in water for a senior person, and appropriate session structure. It also outlines how to adapt each component of the session to accommodate some of the requirements of a senior exerciser.

## How does the ageing process affect our body?

Ageing has a significant effect on the body. The skeletal, muscular, cardiovascular, respiratory and nervous systems are all affected by the ageing process. Some of the changes that occur are outlined in tables 14.1 to 14.4. Age-related changes generally begin to occur at 50 years old, and make their mark at around 65 years old. However, an inactive lifestyle and disuse of the muscles may contribute to the early onset of ageing. Physical activity and

regular use of the muscles can slow down the ageing process, so it is possible for an active 70- or 80-year-old to be in better shape and condition than someone who is inactive and 40. Awareness of age-related changes help you to adapt activities.

## How will movements need to be adapted for the skeletal system?

(*see* Table 14.1 on page 216)
- Movements of the joints will need to be slower and more controlled.
- Excessively high impact activities will place too much stress on joints.
- Emphasis should be placed on working the muscles that will improve posture.
- More joint mobilising activities will be needed.
- Strengthening exercises should be included to improve bone density.
- Further adaptations may need to be made for those with specialist conditions (for example, arthritis, etc.).

| Table 14.1 | The effects of ageing on the skeletal system | |
| --- | --- | --- |
| **Effects of ageing** | | **Associated problems** |
| • Decreased bone density (less calcium in the bones<br>• Calcification (laying down of bone) of the cartilage in joints<br>• Decreased availability of synovial fluid (fluid that lubricates the joints) | | • Brittle bones – osteoporosis<br>• Postural problems such as spinal curvatures<br>• Increased likelihood of joint-associated disease, arthritis etc.<br>• Stiffer and less mobile joints |

| Table 14.2 | The effects of ageing on the muscular system | |
| --- | --- | --- |
| **Effects of ageing** | | **Associated problems** |
| • Decreased motor neurones (nerves transmitting messages to the muscles)<br>• Decreased fast twitch muscle fibres (the fibres used during strength training and power activities)<br>• Decreased concentration of myosin and actin (smallest muscle fibres)<br>• Reduced capillarisation (poorer blood supply to muscles)<br>• Increased connective tissue in the muscles<br>• Reduced elasticity in ligaments and tendons | | • Reduced movement speed<br>• Less potential muscular strength<br>• Loss of muscle tissue<br>• Less potential muscular endurance<br>• Less flexibility<br>• Stiffer and less mobile joints<br>• Weakened pelvic floor muscles |

## How will movements need to be adapted for the muscular system?

(*see* Table 14.2 above)
• All movements will need to be slower.
• More time will need to be allowed for directional changes.
• Movement patterns will need to be sequenced more repeatedly.
• Movements will need to be simpler.
• All activities will need to be less intense.

• Greater emphasis should be placed on alignment and the maintenance of correct technique.
• Explosive movements or high impact moves will be inappropriate.
• A lower number of repetitions of the same exercise will need to be performed, to prevent fatigue.
• Specific activities to strengthen the pelvic floor muscles should be included (discussed in Chapter 15).

| **Table 14.3** | **The effects of ageing on the cardiovascular system** |
|---|---|
| Effects of ageing | Associated problems |
| • Decreased gaseous exchange, elasticity of the lungs and flexibility of the thorax<br>• Lower cardiac output and less efficient circulatory system<br>• Reduced capillary network and less oxygen delivered to the cells<br>• Increased blood pressure | • Reduced oxygen uptake<br>• Lower maximal heart rate and slower recovery rate<br>• Decreased tolerance to fatigue and waste products such as lactic acid<br>• Increased likelihood of disease of the cardiovascular and respiratory system |

| **Table 14.4** | **The effects of ageing on the nervous system** |
|---|---|
| Effects of ageing | Associated problems |
| • Poor short-term memory<br>• Impaired balance<br>• Fewer messages from brain to body due to death of nerve cells | • Forget movement patterns more rapidly<br>• Difficulty stabilising a position and maintaining balance<br>• Reduced body awareness<br>• Reduced movement speed<br>• Increased likelihood of disease of the nervous system (i.e. Parkinson's disease) |

# How will movements need to be adapted for the cardiovascular system?

(*see* Table 14.3 at top of page)
• Activities will need to be less intense.
• Activities may need to be performed for a shorter duration.
• Lower repetitions of intense movements, to prevent fatigue.
• Explosive or high intensity movements will be inappropriate.
• More time will be needed preparing the body for activity, and for recovery afterwards.

• Further adaptations will need to be made for those with specialist conditions (high blood pressure, etc.).

# How will movements need to be adapted for the nervous system?

(*see* Table 14.4 above)
• Movements will need to be simpler.
• Movement patterns will need to be more repetitive, but not excessively so.
• Stable exercise positions will need to be provided.
• Movements will need to be slower.

- Further adaptations will need to be made for those with specialist conditions.

## What are the benefits of water-based activities for the senior participant?

Water provides a highly supportive environment and is an ideal medium for training the older adult. Exercising in water will provide many benefits.

### Buoyancy

- Provides support to the bodyweight and reduces the compression to the weight-bearing joints. This alleviates the stress placed on the joints from normal activities. The joints can relax and any joint pain may be relieved (even if only temporarily). This is especially beneficial for those with joint problems such as arthritis.
- Reduces the impact of jumping movements by 80 per cent when performed at chest depth. It is therefore safe to include modifications of many of the cardiovascular exercises illustrated in Chapter 8.
- Improves the flotation of the body levers and will ease movement of the joints. This will potentially allow them to move through a greater range of motion more comfortably and with less effort. This is especially beneficial for those suffering from arthritis.

### Resistance

- Adds intensity to all movements. Therefore, although water-based exercising is non-weight bearing, the added resistance to movements may be sufficient to stress the bones and lead to improvements in bone density.
- Strengthening of the muscles and other tissues surrounding the joints can improve posture and joint stability.

### Hydrostatic pressure

- Improves the circulation of blood around the body. This is especially beneficial for senior exercisers who generally have a less efficient cardiovascular system.
- Assists the removal of waste products. Again, this is excellent for senior exercisers who are generally less able to tolerate lactic acid (a waste product of anaerobic work).
- Lowers working heart rate. Again, this benefits seniors who will have a lower maximal heart rate.
- Promotes the more effective recovery from exercise. Senior exercisers have a slower recovery rate, but should be able to recover more effectively from water-based training.
- Can help to reduce swelling in the joints.
- Can make it harder to breathe if water is pressing against the ribcage. Exercising in shallower water will be necessary for those who have respiratory problems, or rheumatic diseases that cause fusion of the vertebrae in the thoracic region of the spine.

## Safety considerations for the senior exerciser

Seniors tend to carry higher proportions of body fat, and the density of their bones may be lower. This will make them more buoyant, and will make it more difficult for them to maintain balance in water. Movements will need to be slower and water skills will need to be coached more carefully.

It is essential that seniors are coached how to regain balance if they fall in water. However, they may have less strength to perform the necessary propulsive movements, so it may be necessary for them to exercise in slightly shallower water, although we need to recognise that if such adaptation is needed, the effects of gravity will be increased. Further modification of certain exercises may be needed to ensure they are still safe to perform.

Seniors are more susceptible to feeling the cold and will cool down more quickly. It is a good idea to encourage them to wear swimming caps to reduce heat loss when exercising in water. Exercising in a warmer pool temperature is ideal, and may well be essential for seniors with specialist conditions (arthritis, etc.). However, they can exercise in cooler pools provided they are kept moving to maintain an appropriate temperature, and if the time they spend in the pool is reduced. Long-term regular exercise can help them to maintain body heat more effectively.

Seniors with specialist medical conditions should seek a doctor's permission before they embark on any form of physical activity, as they will need further individual adaptations made to their programme of activities. It is therefore essential that instructors liaise closely with a physiotherapist and a GP to ensure the activities are appropriate. Those wishing to train senior exercisers should enrol on an appropriate training programme.

## How should a seniors programme be structured?

As with all other sessions, sufficient time should be spent warming up before the main activity, and warming down afterwards. A session structure that trains all the fitness components is ideal. A traditional programme format to train all components is outlined in table 8.1 (*see* page 125). A circuit training format that trains all components is outlined in table 12.1 (*see* page 198).

However, the duration and intensity of the whole session and each component will need to be adapted for a seniors programme. The complete session will need to be slightly shorter and of a lower intensity, depending on the fitness of the group. Guidelines for the timing and duration of specialist programmes are outlined in table 5.3 (*see* page 84). More specific guidelines for selecting the appropriate type of activities for a seniors programme are outlined in table 14.5.

| Table 14.5 | Adaptations to session components for a seniors programme |
|---|---|

**Warm-up**
- More mobility exercises for each joint.
- More isolated mobility work for each joint.
- Slower, more controlled mobility exercises that promote an easy but fuller range of motion.
- More mobility exercises for minor joints.
- More emphasis on exercise technique.
- Less intense pulse-raising.
- Fewer directional changes.
- Slower movements.
- Shorter levers.

| Table 14.5 | Adaptations to session components for a seniors programme (cont.) |
|---|---|

## Warm-up
- More advice on how to use water to maintain balance
- Slower transitions
- Fewer stretches
- Easier and more stable, balanced positions
- More care getting into and out of stretch positions

## Cardiovascular
- Spend slightly longer on the re-warmer and cool-down phases, to allow for a more gradual build up and build down of intensity
- Lower intensity maintenance section
- Duration of maintenance should be adapted to suit the ability of the group
- Slower movements
- Fewer explosive moves out of water
- Keep arm movements under the water. Using the arms out of the water may cause a rise in blood pressure
- Use an interval training approach, combining low intensity work with occasional short bursts of moderate intensity activities. The frequency of more moderately paced activities will be dependent on the fitness of the group.

## Muscular strength and endurance
- Fewer repetitions of each exercise
- Lower resistance
- Slower movements through the full range of motion
- Target postural muscles (quadriceps, hamstrings, erector spinae, abdominals, trapezius, calf muscles)
- Target muscles to assist with daily activities: triceps – for pushing out of the bath; biceps – for lifting and carrying objects
- Keep the body immersed and moving throughout to prevent cooling
- Select more stable and comfortable positions
- Include stretches for each muscle once it has finished working. (This will shorten time needed for cooling down.)

## Cool-down
- Shorter component
- Combine stretches with flowing movements to keep warm (i.e. smaller range of motion of stretches)
- Hold static stretches for less time
- Select positions that offer more support and assist balance
- Keep the body immersed and moving throughout to prevent cooling.

# SHORT ANSWER REVISION QUESTIONS

1. State **TWO** age-related physiological changes that occur to the skeletal and muscular systems that will affect exercise.
2. State **TWO** age-related physiological changes that occur to the cardiovascular and nervous system that will affect exercise.
3. State **TWO** ways buoyancy can benefit an older adult group.
4. State how pool temperature may affect programming with an older adult group.
5. Describe the benefits of hydrostatic pressure for the older adult group.
6. List **TEN** specific adaptations to the whole session content and structure that would be appropriate for working with an older adult group

# AQUATIC TRAINING THROUGH PREGNANCY

## 15

## OBJECTIVES

By the end of this session the reader will be able to:

- Identify some of the physiological changes that affect the body during and after pregnancy (ante- and post-natal)
- Recognise some appropriate considerations for adapting the session to work with apparently healthy ante- and post-natal women who have no pregnancy complications and who are used to exercise
- Realise the need for further training in order to work effectively and safely with ante- and post-natal women.

This chapter discusses how the body changes during pregnancy, the benefits of exercising in water for a pregnant woman, and how to structure an ante-natal exercise programme in water.

## How will pregnancy affect the body?

Pregnancy will affect each individual woman slightly differently. However, some key adaptations to the body will affect all women.

### The pelvic floor muscles

These muscles run from the front to the back of the pelvis, forming a 'floor' across the base of the pelvis. When these muscles are weak, urine may leak out when the woman coughs, squats widely, or performs activities that involve jumping. When they are strong it should be possible to cough and jump with legs out to the side (a Jumping Jack) at the same time with no leak of urine. During pregnancy the weight of the baby presses against, and places a stress on, these muscles. During birth an even greater stress is placed on them. Therefore, the inclusion of specific exercises to strengthen the pelvic floor muscles is essential both during and after pregnancy, though everyone can benefit from keeping these muscles strong. (Note: it is also advisable to include these exercises for senior exercisers.)

## NEED TO KNOW

A strengthening exercise for the pelvic floor muscles

1 Sitting, standing or lying.

2 Contract and close the muscles surrounding the back passage, the muscles around the vagina (or penis and scrotum for men), and the muscles around the front passage.

3 Hold the contraction for between 4 and 6 seconds, rest and then repeat a few times.

4 Do not hold the breath.

5 To check that you are performing the exercises correctly and making improvements, try to stop the flow of urine mid-stream. If you can, the muscles are becoming stronger. Note: this should only be checked on one occasion per week.

## The abdominal muscles

The abdominal muscles must stretch and lengthen to accommodate the growing baby. Great care should be taken with any abdominal work when the baby starts to show. Intense abdominal exercises and too much abdominal work at this time can place too much stress on the abdominal muscles, so avoid such activities.

During pregnancy greater emphasis should be placed on contracting the muscles to fixate the spine and maintain correct posture. If the abdominal muscles are stressed, it is possible for them to separate down their mid-line (linea alba). This condition is known post-natally as 'diastasis recti'. (Note: separation of the abdominal muscles is a normal physiological response to pregnancy.) The advice is for participants to

work carefully: generally, it is unlikely that exercise in water would cause overstress.

Once separation has occurred, even greater care is needed for the abdominals: it will be more difficult to regain the figure, and the mother may be left with a permanently rounded tummy. The abdominal muscles should be checked regularly after birth, and any exercise which causes the abdominals to dome should be avoided.

To test for separation of the abdominals:

Lie on the floor with the knees bent, and lift the head. If separation has occurred, a gap may be apparent down the middle of the abdomen. A further check can be provided by placing two fingers widthways into the mid-line of the abdominals, just above or below navel level.

## The pelvis

The pelvic girdle becomes less stable during pregnancy. This is due to the release of a hormone called relaxin that loosens the ligaments around the pelvis in preparation for birth. Any movements involving the pelvis should be either avoided or performed with great care during pregnancy.

Relaxin may also affect other joints such as the knees, fingers, hips and spine. Care must be taken not to exceed the range of motion at any joint, to prevent permanent damage occurring to the ligaments that will result in the joints becoming less stable. It is essential that correct exercise technique is emphasised throughout the ante- or post-natal exercise session.

## The back

The weight of the growing baby will place extra strain on the lumbar spine. This may result in a forward tilt of the pelvis that will cause the lumbar spine to hollow (*see* page 45 for exaggerated lordotic curve). In addition, the centre of gravity will alter and will affect balance. The mother may develop a leaning back posture to counteract these changes, so it is essential that correct posture is coached throughout the session to increase her body awareness. Encouraging the mother to lift the growing baby up and into the pelvis will develop her awareness of correct alignment.

## The cardiovascular system

During pregnancy the volume of blood we pump around the body actually increases, so the heart has to work harder. It therefore adapts and becomes stronger to cope with the demands. Pre-exercise heart rate will be slightly higher during pregnancy due to the increased blood volume and circulatory demands.

High intensity activities may restrict blood flow to the foetus: they should be avoided during pregnancy. It is also wise to exercise for a shorter duration because foetal heart rate may increase if exercise is too prolonged and too intense. Care must also be taken to avoid excessive rises in temperature, which are dangerous to the foetus in the early stages.

## What are the benefits of exercising during pregnancy?

- Decreased aches and pains
- Assistance with weight management
- Easing of constipation
- Improved sleep
- Improved posture
- Improved self-esteem
- Fewer backaches
- Decreased occurrence of varicose veins
- Regaining shape and figure after birth more quickly.

## Why is exercising in water ideal during pregnancy?

**Buoyancy** will provide support to the whole body. The weight of the growing baby will be supported, as will the weight of the growing breasts, so the mother will feel lighter when exercising in water. This additional support provides many benefits for the expectant mother. It will:

- promote relaxation and the release of tension from the muscles that normally have to work to carry the additional body weight
- ease movement through a fuller range of motion without placing the joints under stress
- reduce the weight and stress placed on the pelvic floor muscles
- reduce compression of the joints
- decrease the impact from jumping movements. Therefore, some of the lower intensity cardiovascular exercises illustrated in Chapter 8 can be performed without placing the body at risk
- reduce the stress placed on the pelvic girdle if taking the weight on to one leg
- reduce the stress on the spine during bending and rotating and hip circling movements. (Note: care should still be taken not to exceed a comfortable range of motion, even though this area is more supported. A correct pelvic tilt should also be encouraged.)

**Resistance** provides sufficient intensity to challenge the muscles and maintain their tone, without overworking them. It also reduces the speed of movements, so it is more difficult to exceed a comfortable range of motion.

**Hydrostatic pressure** improves the circulation of blood. It may help to prevent an accumulation of harmful waste products that can potentially cause distress to the foetus.

The **temperature** of the water will have a cooling effect on the body, preventing the body from overheating, something that can be harmful to the foetus. Ensure that rhythmical movements are maintained throughout the session, however, to prevent excessive cooling.

## What are the safety considerations?

It is always advisable to check with a doctor or midwife before starting or continuing an exercise programme when pregnant. Care must be taken to ensure that over-exertion does not occur: the mother should listen to her body and do only what feels comfortable.

In general, during the initial stages of pregnancy, fewer changes will need to be made to the programme for a regular exerciser. However, more precautions will need to be taken during the middle and later stages of pregnancy. In all instances the emphasis should be on maintaining fitness rather than improving fitness while pregnant.

### NEED TO KNOW

When working with pregnant women, exercise should stop and a doctor should be consulted if any of the following occur:

- breathlessness
- excessive colour or pallor
- bleeding from the vagina
- facial expression showing signs of discomfort
- abdominal or chest pain
- sudden swelling of the hands and ankles (oedema)
- excessive fatigue
- feeling faint
- waters break
- extremes of temperature: too hot, too cold
- after class: nausea, vomiting, severe headaches, excessive vaginal discharge, uterine contractions.

# How should the session be structured?

The session should include a warm-up and warm-down. It should aim to maintain rather than develop fitness, so it should contain activities to increase general mobility and improve body awareness. A greater emphasis should be placed on breathing, correct posture and alignment. The duration of the session should be shorter and the intensity much lower. Table 8.1 (*see* page 125) outlines an appropriate structure for training all components of fitness. Specific adaptations to the components of the session are outlined in table 15.1. Note: it is advisable for instructors to consult a midwife when designing specific ante- and post-natal training programmes.

| Table 15.1 | Adaptations to session structure for an ante- and post-natal group |
|---|---|

**Warm-up**
- Emphasise correct posture at the start of, and throughout, the session
- Make movements slower and more controlled
- Increase the number of mobility exercises
- Move all the joints through all possible ranges of motion to reduce stiffness
- Use full range of motion mobility exercises to warm the muscles
- Pulse-raising exercises should be of a much lower intensity, the primary aim being to warm the muscles rather than increase the heart rate
- The intensity of movements should be built up much more gradually to avoid sudden increases in blood pressure
- Directional changes should be minimal to assist maintenance of balance
- Fewer stretches may be needed, especially if full range of motion mobility exercises are included
- Stretch positions should be supported, and care should be taken not to exceed a comfortable range of motion
- The pool wall should be used to assist balance.

**Cardiovascular**
- Work at a much lower intensity for a moderate duration. Aim for a slight breathlessness
- Decrease the number of directional movements; centre of gravity changes making it difficult to balance
- More gradual build-up of intensity to avoid increase in blood pressure
- Fewer jumping moves, to maintain comfort for larger breasts
- Avoid explosive movements that lift the body out of the water
- Use lower impact, rhythmical and free-flowing movements
- Use slower movements and music
- Use simpler and less co-ordinated movement patterns
- Promote full range of motion exercises.

| Table 15.1 | Adaptations to session structure for an ante- and post-natal group (cont.) |
|---|---|

**Muscular strength and endurance**

- Include exercises for the pelvic floor muscles
- No abdominal exercises – be sensitive to amount of fixation of abdominals in water and plan rests
- Select comfortable starting positions
- Avoid exercises that may place excessive pressure on the pelvic girdle
- Use movements related to everyday actions
- Perform fewer repetitions
- Use slower and less intense exercises.

**Cool-down**

- Include range of motion mobility work to maintain a comfortable temperature
- Include specific relaxation work (if water temperature allows)
- Avoid positions that may overstretch the ligaments
- Select balanced and comfortable positions for passive stretching
- Don't hold stretches too long, to maintain rather than develop flexibility.

**Note:** more resting phases should be included throughout the main workout. This can be achieved by including regular periods of free-flowing, rhythmical mobility exercises. If these activities are performed with a staggered foot stance, they will reduce the amount of fixation work needed by the abdominal muscles to maintain balance.

# SHORT ANSWER REVISION QUESTIONS

1. State **THREE** benefits of maintaining active, or exercising, during pregnancy.
2. State **TWO** physiological changes that affect the body during and after pregnancy (ante- and post-natal).
3. Describe the effects of pregnancy on the:
   (a) abdominal muscles.
   (b) pelvic floor muscles.
4. State **TWO** reasons when you would recommend that participation in exercise in water be deferred.
5. Describe how the properties of water may assist movement during pregnancy.
6. State **TEN** adaptations you would make to the overall design and structure of the session for a pregnant group.

# TEACHING, WORKING WITH MUSIC AND CHOREOGRAPHY

# PART FIVE

# TEACHING AN EXERCISE IN WATER SESSION

## OBJECTIVES

By the end of this chapter the reader will be able to:

- Describe some of the qualities of an effective teacher/instructor
- List some of the roles and responsibilities of the teacher/instructor
- State the importance of voice intonation and volume
- State the importance of demonstration
- State the importance of cueing
- Describe different methods of cueing
- State the importance of giving teaching/coaching points
- Recognise a range of visual cues that can be used
- Recognise how the teacher can monitor class performance
- Describe how the teacher can observe and correct individuals
- Discuss the importance of observation and correction
- Recognise how pool structure and design may affect observation and correction
- Discuss an appropriate teaching position for leading exercise in water
- State the limitations of teaching in the pool on observation and correction
- State the benefits of teaching in the pool.

## What are the qualities of a good teacher?

A good teacher should always be friendly, approachable and have concern for the health and safety of participants. They need to have patience, a sense of humour and the ability to motivate, encourage and maintain participants' interest. Listening skills and sensitivity to individual needs are also essential.

## What are the roles of the teacher or instructor?

The main role of the teacher is to plan, teach and evaluate a safe, enjoyable and effective session. Guidelines for planning an exercise in water session are provided in Part 3, Chapters 5–12.

Teachers need to arrive early, before the session is due to start, to prepare equipment and music, screen class participants and make any last-minute safety checks to the environment.

They need to be prepared to adapt the planned session accordingly if there are any unexpected alterations. For example, if the pool temperature is slightly lower than normal, it may be necessary to adapt the session content to ensure participants are kept sufficiently warm.

Teachers will need to introduce themselves to new participants, and encourage individuals to communicate their personal fitness goals and any special requirements. They should be confident and able to deal with any special requirements that are identified to them. Alternatively, if they are not qualified to deal with the needs of a participant, they should refer them to the appropriate person, for example a doctor.

They will also need to maintain control of the class before, during and after the session, ensuring participants enter the pool in a controlled and appropriate manner, and familiarise themselves with the depth of the water. Control should be maintained throughout the session by giving clear and accurate instructions and demonstrations, including advance cueing of each activity. During the session, the teacher should be vigilant and monitor class performance, giving coaching advice to improve the performance of participants when needed. They should also encourage the class when they perform an exercise particularly well, or adapt an exercise if a participant is struggling or unable to perform a specific movement.

When the session is finished, the teacher should thank participants for attending, encourage them to leave the pool in a controlled manner and invite questions. Any equipment used should be packed away safely. Teachers need to be prepared to stay slightly later than the scheduled duration of the class to meet these requirements.

The teacher will also need to reflect on the class they have taught. Were the planned components safe and effective? Could everyone cope with the activities? Was the music of a correct pace? Could the class follow their instructions and demonstrations? How did they manage to observe and correct performance? What changes need to be made to improve future sessions? Evaluating one's performance is often not an easy task; it can be useful to seek further feedback from participants and, on occasion, employers and other teachers.

## How can the teacher communicate effectively with the class?

The primary aim of the teacher is to communicate with the class.

There are two main ways of communicating this information:

1 **Visually** through demonstrations and body language
2 **Verbally** through spoken instructions.

### NEED TO KNOW

Participants need to know:
- what exercise they should be doing (instructions)
- when they should be doing it (cueing – visual and verbal)
- how they should be doing it (teaching points)
- how to adapt the exercise to meet their needs; if they cannot do it they need to be shown alternatives
- how to make the exercise harder to provide more of a challenge as their fitness and skill level improves (progressions).

The combined usage of both visual and verbal communication techniques is usually the most effective, since people learn in different ways. To adopt one single teaching style over another can reduce one's overall effectiveness as a teacher. However, there are further issues to consider that will maximise the effectiveness of these strategies.

## How will voice volume and intonation affect communication?

Verbal communication requires the voice to be loud and clear. A voice that is too quiet will not be heard, especially in the pool environment where acoustics are notoriously bad. It may also infer that the instructor is timid and lacks confidence. Alternatively, shouting will distort the sound of the voice and can make the instructor appear aggressive. Therefore, it is necessary for the instructor to find a way of modulating their voice so that it is audible and establishes control.

The intonation of the voice is also important. Monotone voices can become uninteresting, and will provide no emphasis to key coaching points. The voice intonation should therefore be varied to emphasise the key instructions and safety advice being given. Tone of voice can also be varied to reflect the atmosphere of the specific component of the session. It should be used to encourage in components where participants are required to work harder (cardiovascular and muscular strength and endurance training), and should be softer during relaxation and stretching components of the session.

| Table 16.1 | Suggested visual cue signs |
|---|---|
| Move forward | Pull the palms of the hands towards the body to indicate that the group should move towards you. |
| Move back | Push the palms away from the body to indicate that the group should move away from you. |
| Move right or left | Point strongly to the right or left and look towards the direction of travel. |
| Turn | Raise the arm in the air and draw a circle to indicate a full turn, or a semi-circle to indicate half a turn. |
| Stop | Raise the hand with the palm away from your body and elbow extended to indicate stop. (This is useful for controlling large circuits.) |
| Make moves smaller | Raise the hand in front of you, elbow extended, and place the forefinger and thumb an inch apart to indicate that the movement should be made smaller. Alternatively, with the arm extended and the palm facing the floor, the arm can be moved down to indicate that the intensity should be brought down. |
| Perform exercise in neutral mode | Place the hands on top of the shoulders to indicate that the exercise should be performed in neutral mode, with the shoulders under water. Demonstrate the exercise with no rebounding motion. |

| Table 16.1 | Suggested visual cue signs (cont.) |
| --- | --- |
| Perform exercise in suspend mode | With palms facing upwards, lift the arms up and then use the arms to mimic the movement of the legs. Ideally, if there are steps available, perform the exercise holding the steps so the feet are off the floor. |
| Perform exercise in rebound mode | Demonstrate the movement in a bouncier style and use the hands to show the body lifting and lowering through the water. |

Note: The visual cue signs above are only suggestions, and certainly not compulsory. Each teacher will find their own methods for controlling movement of the class.

## How will the clarity of instruction affect communication?

Instructions need to be spoken at an appropriate pace and in a concise and precise manner to maximise their effectiveness. If instructions are rushed, they may appear garbled and it is more than likely they will be misunderstood. The vocabulary used should be recognisable by participants for ease of understanding. If they do not know the names of the exercises they are supposed to perform, they will not follow effectively. However, lengthy explanations will be tedious and participants will lose interest. This is when it is most useful to use visual coaching strategies.

## How will visual cueing enhance communication?

Visual cues are gestures of the body. Gesturing movements of the arms can indicate the direction of movement. Gesturing movements of the fingers and hand can be used to show how many times the exercise should be performed, cue a new move, indicate a turn in the movement and show correct hand position. Facial expressions can be used to encourage the class (e.g. smiling). A combination of these skills will assist with class control and motivation.

However, too many gestures may become irritating and hard to follow. In addition, the gestures used need to be consistent so that the participants know what is expected of them. If visual cues are used, they need to be strong and clear; small and weak visual signals do not provide effective control.

## How can demonstrations be used to improve class performance?

A swift demonstration of a movement allows the teacher to show exactly how the body should move, and in which direction. However, it is essential that their body alignment and exercise technique are precise and accurate, and that the speed of their demonstration accurately reflects the buoyancy and resistance of the water. A poor demonstration will be ineffective, since participants will have to interpret the exercise in their own way and may subsequently perform unsafely or ineffectively.

When demonstrating an exercise, the teacher should be in full view of all participants. Positioning themselves in a place where participants can see clearly, without having to turn around, is best. In addition, it is essential that the body is fully visible during demonstrations. Baggy clothing is not appropriate. It will restrict participants' observation of the moving joints, requiring them to make their own interpretation of the movement being performed.

For movements that are very complex, it is advisable to demonstrate and allow participants to perform a dry run to check they can perform the movement prior to its inclusion in a specific movement routine. However, the class should be kept moving to keep them warm and maintain the intensity of the workout. An alternative approach is to use the choreography techniques with visual previews and holding patterns (*see* Chapter 17). This approach allows complex movement patterns to be built up gradually, without interrupting the continuity of the session.

## Where should the teacher be positioned to demonstrate and observe the class?

Some teachers prefer to teach their sessions from the deck, whereas others prefer to teach in the water. The key advantage of teaching from the deck is that the teacher is able to scan the group quickly and move around to assist individuals. They are more likely to observe a struggling participant and can quickly call for help from the lifeguard, or provide their own rescue techniques if working on the deck. In addition, it is much easier for them to be seen clearly by the class. However, a disadvantage of teaching from the poolside is that the instructor will be performing

in a more hazardous environment. Safety issues regarding poolside are discussed in Chapter 4.

The main advantage of teaching in the pool is that the teacher will be able to demonstrate the exercise at an appropriate speed, and their movements will be supported by the water. Unfortunately, the biggest disadvantage is that participants will not be able to see what the teacher is doing and can only follow their verbal instructions. Teaching in the pool is perhaps only acceptable practice if the participants are regular attendees, are familiar with the instructions used by the teacher and know how all exercises should be performed. However, as verbal instructions are the only method used, the teacher is potentially limiting their communication with the group. A further disadvantage is that the teacher will not be able to move around the pool to observe and control direction changes so effectively.

While poolside teaching is considered best practice, teachers should not be restricted and should feel able to enter the pool if it will help them to assist the performance of their class or a class member. However, if working in the pool restricts teaching opportunities, it should not be used. Teaching from the deck provides no guarantee that participants will be observed, corrected and encouraged sufficiently, although it perhaps provides greater opportunity for this to occur.

## How can the teacher monitor and correct participants' performance?

During land-based classes, it is recommended that the teacher frequently moves among the class to correct technique. Obviously, this is not possible during a water-based session. The teacher should therefore adopt the alternative strategy of changing class front. Teaching from different sides of the pool will allow different participants to be positioned at the front of the class, and will thus improve the teacher's observation of them. In addition, occasional and careful movement around the poolside can help the instructor to observe and interact more closely with individual participants.

However, it is still relatively difficult to see what participants are doing due to the refraction caused by the water. Refraction distorts vision through water and creates an optical illusion. Therefore, participants' movements will be slightly distorted. It is therefore essential that frequent reminders of correct posture and joint alignment are provided to ensure participants perform safely. Advising participants how they should feel, telling them which muscles they should feel working and asking for feedback are other strategies for monitoring performance. This provides the instructor with an opportunity to accommodate individuals by offering alternative exercises, advice on how to use the water, and advice on how to perform each activity for maximal effectiveness.

## SHORT ANSWER REVISION QUESTIONS

1. List **FIVE** qualities of an effective teacher/instructor.
2. State **FOUR** roles and responsibilities of the teacher/instructor.
3. State the importance of
    (a) voice intonation and volume:
    (b) demonstration
    (c) cueing.
4. Describe verbal cueing.
5. Describe visual cueing.
6. Describe how body language affects communication.
7. State **TWO** reasons for giving teaching/coaching points.
8. Describe **TWO** visual cues and when they can be used.
9. State the importance of observation and correction.
10. Describe **TWO** ways the teacher can correct and assist individual performance.
11. Discuss the importance of teaching position.
12. State **TWO** pool-related factors that may affect observation of the class and teaching position.
13. State **TWO** reasons why teaching on the poolside is preferred over teaching in the water.
14. Give **TWO** reasons when it may be appropriate to teach in the water.

# WORKING WITH MUSIC AND CHOREOGRAPHY

17

## OBJECTIVES

By the end of this chapter the reader will be able to:

- State some advantages and disadvantages of using music in a water-based session
- Recognise factors that will affect working to the beat and phrase in water
- Recognise appropriate music speed for different components
- Describe different ways music can be used
- Describe basic methods of varying chorography
- Recognise music licences needed to play music in a water-based session.

The use of music for the water-based workout is optional and should only be used if the participants enjoy working with music. The teacher needs to be skilled at using music and must possess the necessary music licences (PPL and PRS), or subscribe to music agencies that pre-record tapes and include a subscription fee that is paid to the appropriate licensing body.

## Why use music?

Most people enjoy listening to music, and many enjoy actually exercising to music. Music is fun and can enhance both the atmosphere created and the performance of participants. Some of the advantages and disadvantages of using music are listed in table 17.1.

## Is it possible to work to the beat and phrase of the music in water?

There is much controversy surrounding working to the music when exercising in water, the primary issue being whether it is possible for everyone to work to the same beat and phrase of the music when immersed in water.

Opponents to working to the beat and phrase of the music suggest that it is not possible to dictate a 'one speed for all' approach because individuals have different body types, different body compositions, carry body fat in different areas and are of different fitness levels. Therefore, they need to exercise at their own pace. This is totally accurate; however, it is equally an issue during land-based activities. On land, different body types are accommodated by offering alternative exercises.

Sometimes, it is necessary to offer a totally

different exercise for the same body part to enable participants to continue working out safely and effectively. This can also be practised in water. The lists of progressions for all the exercises illustrated at the end of Chapters 6–11 are intended as a guide for selecting an appropriate intensity for different abilities.

Interestingly enough, synchronised swimmers manage to work effectively to both the beat and phrase of the music, even though their routines are performed in very deep water where this is much harder to achieve. This is perhaps because they are skilful at manipulating the water, skilful at using the music, and are of a comparatively leaner body composition than non-exercisers.

It is therefore suggested that if the participants are sufficiently skilled at using the water, and of an appropriate fitness level and body composition, then the teacher should encourage work to the beat and phrase of the music. However, it is often the beat of the music that dictates the speed. Therefore, selecting an appropriate speed of music is essential. Guidelines for appropriate music speed ranges for different components of the session are outlined in table 17.2, page 238.

Alternatively, if the participants are not skilled at using the water, are less fit and are carrying a higher proportion of body fat, this may not be appropriate. Therefore, the instructor should aim to cue each change of movement sequence to the phrase, but allow participants to work at a pace that suits them. It may be necessary to allow more time for them to perform each activity. Therefore, changes to movement patterns will need to be less frequent. In addition, alternative exercises may need to be provided to assist their performance, as will plenty of advice on how to manipulate the water and perform propulsive movements. The music selected for specialist groups, the less fit and persons with a higher percentage of body fat should be of a slower pace. This will allow them to perform more of the activities to the beat dictated by the music.

A personal recommendation is that teachers should possess the skill and ability to cue movements to the music phrase. However, they should allow and positively encourage participants to work at a pace (beat) that suits their requirements. From experience, it is often the participants who are unable to manipulate water effectively who cannot maintain work to the musical phrasing.

| **Table 17.1** | **The advantages and disadvantages of using music in an exercise in water session** |
|---|---|
| Advantages of using music | Disadvantages of using music |
| <ul><li>Creates a fun atmosphere for participants and adds interest</li><li>Routines can be choreographed to different themes to add greater fun and socialisation, for example using circles and partner work</li><li>Motivates the class</li><li>Assists control of group by dictating pace</li><li>Assists planning of the session</li><li>Adds enjoyment to the session.</li></ul> | <ul><li>May create inappropriate atmosphere for desired component</li><li>Can de-motivate if people do not like the music chosen</li><li>Can over-motivate and encourage participants to work too hard when they are tired</li><li>Can dictate an inappropriate pace (too fast or too slow) so that participants are unable to keep up or achieve effective transitions in the water between moves.</li></ul> |

| Table 17.1 | The advantages and disadvantages of using music in an exercise in water session (cont.) |
|---|---|
| Advantages of using music | Disadvantages of using music |
| • Can be a cost-effective investment, adding motivation and interest. | • Can be too loud so that participants may not be able to hear the teacher, or too quiet, which may detract from enjoyment<br>• Poor acoustics will also have an effect on the sound of the music<br>• Sensitivity to other pool users must also be considered<br>• If the teacher has not planned alternatives, or is not prepared to adapt, it may make the session too rigid<br>• Can be monotonous or boring if an insufficient variety of music is used to accommodate different tastes<br>• Tapes, music licences and audio equipment such as head microphones are expensive<br>• Some people actually prefer not to exercise with music!<br>• Pool environment and humidity will affect the equipment and quality of tapes. |

| Table 17.2 | Guidelines for selecting music of an appropriate speed |
|---|---|
| Component of the session | Approximate guidelines for the speed of music |
| Warming up (mobility, pulse-raising and preparatory stretch and re-warmer) | 120–130 beats per minute (bpm) |
| Aerobic component | 125–135 bpm |
| Resistance training | 120–125 bpm |
| Step training | 120–125 bpm |
| Post-workout stretching | 110–125 bpm |
| Relaxation | 80–110 bpm |
| Re-vitalise | 120–125 bpm |

# What is an appropriate music speed?

Most movements will need to be performed at half time in water. For example, on land a Jumping Jack (illustrated in Chapter 8) will take two counts of music to perform the complete movement. In water, the same exercise will take four counts to complete (this is for a person with an average body composition and fitness level working to a speed of music between 120–135 bpm). Obviously, exercises that require a larger range of motion to be performed will take longer than an exercise that works through a smaller range of motion. Therefore, careful consideration needs to be given both to the movements and the music speed selected to ensure appropriate variations of speed can be made for exercises to be executed effectively.

Additionally, the speed of music selected will be dependent on the water depth, the activity and the skill, fitness and body composition of participants. Leaner participants, persons skilled at using water and fitter participants will generally be able to move at a slightly faster tempo, whereas less fit participants, specialist groups, curvaceous body types, and people less skilled at using water will need to work at a slower pace. When exercising in deep water, the pace of the music may need to be slower; if this is the case, working to the beat and phrase of the music is less essential.

A guideline for appropriate music speeds for different components of the session is outlined in table 17.2. However, it is emphasised that the speeds suggested are only a guideline. Some people may need to work more slowly and some may be able to perform faster. It is a good idea for a teacher to practise moves in the water to see how effectively they work to different music speeds. However, they need to appreciate that their own body composition may allow them to perform some of the exercises more or less effectively than persons with a different body composition and body type. Teachers should seek constant feedback from their participants, to check they are able to move at the speed being dictated.

# How can music be used?

## Background

This is where music is played, but the movements are not executed in time to the music, nor are any changes in movement cued to the music phrase. This approach is traditionally adopted during a circuit-training component and in the relaxation component of the session. Music can also be used in the background for deep-water training.

## Beat and phrasing

This is where any changes of a movement sequence are planned to occur at the start of a phrase, and the movements are also performed (ideally) to the beat of the music. It is acceptable if people less skilled at using the water, and more buoyant body types, change movements to the musical phrase, but perform at a pace (beat) that suits their ability and requirements. This approach is traditionally used during muscular strength and endurance training. It can also be used during the warm-up and cardiovascular components, as well as in components using equipment when choreography is minimal.

## Verse and chorus choreography

This is where the music is broken down and the verse and chorus identified. A sequence of movements is planned to be performed and repeated for the verse and another sequence of movements is planned to be repeated for the chorus. All changes of movement should occur to the phrase of the music. This approach can be ideal when working with those less skilled at using the water. If the exercises selected are simple, and changes to movements are less frequent, participants can work effectively and stay working to the music phrase. Each participant may need to work at a slightly different pace. This approach is traditionally used in the cardiovascular component. It can also work effectively in the warm-up and cool-down components.

## Add-on choreography

In its most simplistic form, add-on choreography is about adding one move to another move. For example: one move (Jumping Jacks, 32 counts) is performed for a set number of counts or until it has been mastered by the group. Another move is then performed (Jogging forwards, 16 counts, and back, 16 counts). The two moves are then added together to provide a complete movement sequence. Once this sequence has been learned, the repetitions of each movement can be reduced and performed to a specific phrase of the music (pyramid technique). This technique can be repeated with a new series of movements. The repetitions of the second sequence of movements can also be reduced and broken down using a pyramid technique to form a second movement sequence. The two sequences can then be added together and performed until the group is competent at performing the two sequences. A third series of movements can then be taught, broken down and added on to the first and second sequences.

The number of movement sequences that can be broken down and added together will depend on the skills and fitness of the group and the complexity of the movements. This approach to choreography is traditionally used in the cardiovascular training component. It can also work effectively in the warm-up.

**NB**: For instructors and teachers who prefer working to music, a range of other choreography techniques that can be used in a water-based session are discussed in the *Complete Guide to Exercise to Music*.

## How can choreography be broken down?

There are a number of ways in which choreography can be broken down to assist learning.

## Holding patterns and visual previews

A holding pattern is a movement that the class can perform while the teacher demonstrates and provides a visual preview of the next development or progression of that move.

For example:
**Holding pattern**: Class performs 2 Sploosh and 4 Jogs facing the front (16 counts).
**Visual preview**: Teacher demonstrates Sploosh with half turn to face back and then front of pool again, so that a full circle of Splooshes is performed (16 counts).
**Holding pattern**: Class performs a series of Jumping Jacks.
**Visual preview**: Teacher demonstrates Leap Frogs or Jacks travelling forwards or backwards.

See tables 17.3 and 17.4 for suggestions on how to develop basic choreography movements.

## Pyramid

A pyramid is where the number of repetitions of an exercise or sequence of exercises is reduced sequentially to make up the final sequence or combination.

**For example:**

1 × 32 counts Jumping Jacks

1 × 32 counts Jogging: forwards 16 counts and backwards 16 counts

Reduce pyramid to 1 × 16 counts for each movement listed above

Reduce pyramid to 1 × 8 counts for each movement listed above

A variation of pyramiding can be to increase rather than decrease the repetitions. This can increase the intensity and endurance required.

**For example:**

Jog forwards 8 counts

Jacks 8 counts

Jog back 8 counts

Leap Frogs 8 counts

Repeat all for 16 counts each

Repeat all for 32 counts each

A further variation is to work both up and down the pyramid.

**For example (using the example moves above):**

All moves for 8 counts

All moves for 16 counts

All moves for 32 counts

All moves for 16 counts

All moves for 8 counts

## How can choreography be varied?

There are only a certain number of directions in which our joints can move. In addition, most travelling movements require specific propulsive arm movements to create and assist with movement. These factors will affect the choreography. However, they need not limit choreography ideas. Constantly looking for new movements is often time-consuming and not always successful. It is more effective to find ways of varying the movements we already use. This can be achieved by:

- putting different movement combinations together to form a sequence
- varying the speed of the movements in a sequence (i.e. slow, slow, quick, quick, slow)
- moving the sequence in a different direction (forwards, backwards, sideways, to a diagonal, in a circle)
- varying the arm line (breast stroke or side raises) and hand position (slice, cup or open)
- changing the length of the lever (half lever knee raise or full leg kick)
- using a turn to vary the body part leading the move (for example, run forwards through the water, half turn and run backwards through the water in the same direction)
- performing more or fewer repetitions of a specific movement while still allowing for effective performance
- performing an exercise or part of a sequence of exercises in a different exercise mode (neutral, rebound or suspended)
- performing a sequence of movements in a different pattern around the pool (circles, Figure Eights, lines or in a circuit format)
- changing the exercise mode – rebound, suspend, neutral.

## Exercise modes

Most movements can be performed in one of three modes:

1  Rebounding mode, where the body lifts up and down through the water each time.
2  Neutral mode, where the shoulders stay under the water and the movement is completed without lifting out of the water.
3  Suspended and buoyant mode, where the

movement is performed but the feet do not touch the floor. This can be very intense and should only be used in the main workout. Tables 17.3 and 17.4 provide specific exam- ples of how some of these choreography tools can be applied to the basic choreography moves.

| Table 17.3 | Application of choreography tools to basic choreography | | |
|---|---|---|---|
| Choreography tools | Jog | Jumping Jacks | Sploosh |
| Lever length | High knee Jog, or heel to buttocks Jog | Leap Frogs | Tuck Jumps |
| ROM | Rebound Neutral Suspend | Rebound Neutral Suspend | Rebound Neutral Suspend |
| Rhythm | Slow, slow, quick, quick, quick, quick | 1 Slow – rebound 2 Quick – neutral | Sploosh x 2 Jog x 4 |
| Travel | Forwards or backwards | Travel forwards or backwards | Back Kicks travelling backwards |
| Turn | 4 forward, half turn and repeat in square | 8 Jacks, turn and repeat | Sploosh x 2, Jog x 4 with half or full turn on Sploosh |

| Table 17.4 | Application of choreography tools to basic choreography | | |
|---|---|---|---|
| Choreography tools | Rocking Horse | Side Squats | Flick Kicks |
| Lever length | Full knee extension at front and rear | Use longer arm lever to pull water | Raise the knees higher and extend the knee |
| ROM | Rebound Neutral | Rebound Gazelles Neutral travel | Rebound Neutral |

| Table 17.4 | Application of choreography tools to basic choreography (cont.) | | |
|---|---|---|---|
| Choreography tools | Rocking Horse | Side Squats | Flick Kicks |
| Rhythm | Forwards 2 counts and backwards 2 counts<br>4 single rocks forward and backwards | 1 Slow Side Squat 2 Quick Gazelle Leaps; repeat same direction | Single kick right and left (slow). Double kick right (quick). Repeat left leg leading |
| Travel | Travel forwards, full length of pool | Vary travel to diagonal corners | Travel backwards with arm push. Lean body types may be able to travel forwards if arms pull water strongly |
| Turn | Travel forwards 8 – turn to face other direction | 2 Side Squats. 4 Jogs with half turn to face back. Repeat travelling in same direction. Move back in other direction | Travel back, half turn and repeat a backwards square |

# SHORT ANSWER REVISION QUESTIONS

1. State **TWO** advantages of using music in a water-based session.
2. State **TWO** disadvantages of using music in a water-based session.
3. List **THREE** factors that will affect working to the beat and phrase in water.
4. Describe an appropriate music speed and choice for:
   (a) the warm-up element in a water-based session
   (b) cardiovascular training in a water-based session
   (c) MSE in a water-based session
   (d) the cool-down in a water-based session
   (e) a circuit-style water-based session.
5. State **THREE** ways music can be used in a water-based session.
6. State **FOUR** ways basic choreography and movements can be varied in a water-based session.
7. Name **TWO** companies who specialise in preparing music for use in fitness classes (if in doubt, see useful addresses section).

# LESSON PLANS

18

This chapter provides a variety of lesson plans that can be used for water-based training. Each of the following tables will provide you with some ideas for planning different components of the session and using different approaches. As you become more confident in the instructor/teacher role, you will be able to adapt them to your own preferences.

| Table 18.1 | General warm-up – mobility, pulse-raising and preparatory stretches | | |
|---|---|---|---|
| Music Counts | Exercise | Adaptation | Progression |
| 32 | **A** <br> Light Jog in place | Slower pace | Higher knees |
| 16 | **B** <br> Jumping Jacks with breaststroke arms | Open fingers or slice | Pull water harder <br> Rebound |
| 16 | **C** <br> Spotty Dogs | Slice arms <br> Slower pace | Pull water harder <br> Lengthen stride |
| 32 | Repeat B & C | Cold pool – repeat again | |
| 16 right <br> 16 left <br> 32 both | **D** <br> Figure Eight shoulder mobility. Add shoulder girdle, draw forwards and back. Final set of 16 | Slice water <br> Open fingers <br> Staggered stance <br> Straddle stance <br> Slower move | Stronger push <br> Faster move |
| 96 | Repeat B, C and D <br> Build intensity | As above | As above |

| Table 18.1 | General warm-up - mobility, pulse-raising and preparatory stretches (cont.) | | |
|---|---|---|---|
| Music Counts | Exercise | Adaptation | Progression |
| 32 | E<br>Bear Hugs<br>Mobilise shoulders<br>and ROM Chest and<br>Middle Back stretch | Slower and smaller<br>Static stretch | Fuller ROM |
| 16<br>16<br>16<br>16 | F<br>Side Squats right<br>Spotty Dogs<br>Side Squats left<br>Spotty Dogs | Smaller stride<br>Slice water | Stronger pull<br>Rebound |
| 16<br>16<br>32 | G<br>Run forwards<br>Kick backwards<br>Jumping Jacks | Slower move<br>Open fingers | Pull water harder<br>Kick water harder<br>Rebound |
| 4 × 32 | Repeat F & G | No repeat if water warm | |
| 32 | H<br>Jog heels to bottom<br>Mobilise knees and<br>ROM<br>Front of thigh stretch | Smaller range of<br>motion<br>Static front of<br>thigh stretch | Stronger Jog and push<br>water |
| 16<br>16 | I<br>Jog high knees<br>Static hamstring<br>Stretch right and left | Float leg and scull with<br>both arms<br>Hold poolside | Lift leg higher. Scull |
| 16 | J<br>Static tricep stretch | Without movement | With Jog |
| 32 | Jog to poolside<br>Static calf stretch | Use partners if pool<br>wall space limited | Foot against wall for<br>calf stretch |

Note: Aim to increase intensity at each repeat according to group ability.

| Table 18.2 (a) | Cardiovascular training | | |
|---|---|---|---|
| Music Counts | Exercise | Adaptation | Progression |
| 16 | **A** Run forwards | Slower Jog | Stronger pull |
| 16 | **B** Kick Flick backwards | | Kick harder |
| 32 | **C** Jumping Jacks | | Rebound |
| 32 | Repeat A & B | | |
| 32 | **D** Ballet Jump | Jumping Jacks | Jump Higher |
| 32 | Repeat A & B | | |
| 32 | **E** Leap Frog | Smaller jump | Jump higher |
| 64 | Repeat A, B & D | | |
| 64 | Repeat A, B & D | | |
| 64 | **G** Farmer Giles | Smaller ROM | Extend lever – kick |
| 64 | **H** Rocking Horse Right leg leads Face right side | Keep knee bent Smaller ROM Open fingers | Extend lever – kick Rebound Stronger push |
| 128 | Repeat G to front Repeat H to left | | |
| 16 | **A** Run forwards | Slower jog | Stronger pull |
| 16 | **B** Kick Flick backwards | | Kick harder |

| Table 18.2 (a) | Cardiovascular training (cont.) | | |
|---|---|---|---|
| Music Counts | Exercise | Adaptation | Progression |
| 32 | D<br>Ballet Jump | Jumping Jacks/Sploosh | Jump Higher |
| 128 | Repeat G & H<br>Right leg leads<br>then left | | |
| 16 | A<br>Run forwards | Slower Jog | Stronger pull |
| 16 | B<br>Kick backwards | | Kick backwards |
| 32 | E<br>Leap Frog | Smaller jump | Jump higher |
| 128 | Repeat G & H<br>Right leg leads<br>then left | | |

| Table 18.2 (b) | Jogging – interval heart rate training | | |
|---|---|---|---|
| Set up: Explain RPE scale 0–10 | | | |
| Music Counts | Exercise | Adaptation | Progression |
| 5 minutes | Jog technique | N.B. Individual chooses own perceived level of | |
| 1 minute | Jog RPE 4o | exertion on the RPE scale. They can increase | |
| 30 seconds | Jog RPE 6o | or decrease pace accordingly. | |
| Total 6 minutes | Repeat × 4 | | |
| 30 seconds | Jog RPE 5 | | |
| 15 seconds | Jog RPE 8 | | |
| Toal 4 minutes | Repeat × 4 | | |

| Table 18.2 (c) | Aim to hold heart rate in training zone |
| --- | --- |

**Set up:** Group forms two concentric circles (inside and outside circle)
Same number of people in each circle
Face partner in opposite circle
Label partners A and B

| Music Counts | Exercise | Adaptation | Progression |
| --- | --- | --- | --- |
| 32 | Jog in place | Smaller jump | Higher jump |
| 32<br>Chorus | **A**<br>As jump out of water. When As land, Bs jump out of water. Repeat | | |
| 64<br>Verse | **B**<br>Run in full circle. Outer circle clockwise, inner circle anti-clockwise | | |
| 32s<br>Instrumental (1) | **C**<br>Cross hands with partner and spin right then left | | |
| 32<br>Instrumental (2) | **D**<br>Farmer Giles | | |
| | Repeat A, B, C & D to respective verse/chorus pattern approx 4 times | | |

| Table 18.2 (d) | Aim to hold heart rate in training zone | | |
|---|---|---|---|
| Music Counts | Exercise | Adaptation | Progression |
| 16 | A<br>Run forwards | Slower Jog | Faster pace |
| 16 | B<br>Half turn to face right and 4 Side Squats away from front | | |
| 32 | Repeat A & B above with half turn left | | |
| 64 | C<br>Sploosh with half turn after each 16 counts | Smaller jump<br>Leave out turn | Larger jump |
| 16 | D<br>Run forwards | | |
| 16 | E<br>Half-turn and 4 Side Squats | | |
| 32 | F<br>Sploosh with half turn right after each one | | |
| 64 | Repeat D, E and F with half turn left | | |
| 32 | G<br>Run into square 4 to front, 4 to right, 4 to back, 4 to left | | |
| 32 | Repeat G to opposite side | | |

| Table 18.2 (d) | Aim to hold heart rate in training zone (cont.) | | |
|---|---|---|---|
| Music Counts | Exercise | Adaptation | Progression |
| 16 | **H**<br>Ballet Jumps | Sploosh | Higher Jump |
| 32 | Repeat G to right | | |
| 16 | Repeat H | | |
| 32 | **I**<br>4 Gazelle Leaps right and 4 left | Side Squats | |
| 32 | Repeat I | | |
| 16 | **J**<br>Leap Frogs | Smaller jump | Higher jump |
| 32 | **K**<br>4 Gazelle Leaps right and Leap Frogs | | |
| 32 | Repeat K | | |

## Table 18.2 (e)  Aim to hold heart rate in training zone (Fish and Chips)

**Set up**: Group forms four lines

Tutor gives each participant the label of either Fish or Chips

Group performs same exercise on tutor command from following list

**Exercise commands:**

- Ballet Jumps          40 seconds then front person runs to back
- Jump Jacks           40 seconds then front person runs to back
- Sploosh             40 seconds then front person runs to back
- Leap Frogs          40 seconds then front person runs to back

1 and 2 swap lines
3 and 4 swap lines

Repeat above commands with different exercises.

At any point the tutor can shout fish and chips (together or separate), at which point all participants with that label run to the designated end of pool. When everyone is at the end of the pool, they return to the starting place. Meanwhile, other participants continue the exercise command specified.

**Fish and Chips – Lined and Command circuit**

|  | 1 ⟷ | 2 | 3 ⟷ | 4 |
|------|------|------|------|------|
|  | XF | XF | XF | XF |
| Fish | XC | XC | XC | XC |
|  | Chips |  |  |  |
|  | XF | XF | XF | XF |
|  | XC | XC | XC | XC |

| Table 18.2 (f) | Cool down: aim to hold heart rate then lower out of training zone | | |
|---|---|---|---|
| Set up: | Group forms one circle<br>Label partners A and B<br>Face partner in opposite direction of circle<br>(A – clockwise/B – anti-clockwise) | | |
| Music Counts | Exercise | Adaptation | Progression |
| 32 | Jog in place | Slower Jog | Faster pace |
| 16 | Farmer Giles | Smaller ROM | Kick water harder<br>Extend lever |
| 32 | Daisy chain in a circle. Pass around the circle joining right hand to partner's right hand, then left hand to left. Move in a full circle back to partner | | |
| 16<br>16 | Link arms and spin right<br>Link arms and spin left | Jog in place | |
| 32 | Back to back (hoe down) | Kick in place | |
| 144 x 4 | Repeat above x 4<br>Lower intensity as per group needs | | |

| Table 18.3 (a) | Muscular endurance and low intensity cardiovascular workout |
|---|---|

**Set up:** Two rows or half split circuit approach

Row 1 XXXXXXXXXXXXXXXXXXXXXXXXXXXXX perform cardio move

Row 2 XXXXXXXXXXXXXXXXXXXXXXXXXXXXX perform MSE move

| Example of cardio moves | Example of MSE |
|---|---|
| Jumping Jacks | Push-ups |
| Sploosh | Scissor Legs |
| Shoot Ball | Abdominal pull through |

Time can vary for each exercise from 30 seconds to 60 seconds depending on fitness
Group continually changes sides of pool to complete all exercises

| Table 18.3 (b) | Muscular endurance and low intensity cardiovascular workout with woggles |
|---|---|

**Set up:** Jog in circle to collect woggles, change direction to resist eddy currents. Find space and perform. On completion, Jog in circle to return woggles.

| Music Counts | Exercise | Adaptation | Progression |
|---|---|---|---|
| 1 minute | Woggle is held in front of the body, knees lift to touch woggle Jog lift knees to woggle | Slower ROM | Faster pace |
| 1 minute | Chest Press woggle | Slower move | Stronger push |
| 2 minutes | Repeat | | |

| Table 18.3 (b) | Muscular endurance and low intensity cardiovascular workout with woggles (cont.) | | |
|---|---|---|---|
| Music Counts | Exercise | Adaptation | Progression |
| 1 minute | Woggle is held in front of body, kick to touch woggle<br>Jog kick woggles | Just knees | Rebound |
| 1 minute | Tricep pushdown | Just press hands | Knot woggle |
| 2 minutes | Repeat | | |
| 1 minute | Jacks and squeeze | | |
| 1 minute | Ski press | Slower pace | Rebound |
| 2 minutes | Repeat | | |
| 1 minute | Jack and reverse squeeze | No woggle | Rebound |
| 1 minute | Woggle Flyes | Slower pace | Faster pace |
| 2 minutes | Repeat | | |
| 1 minute | Scissor legs | Poolside balance | Increase pace |
| 1 minute | Breaststroke legs | Poolside balance | Squeeze woggle while scissoring |
| 1 minute | Leg kicks | Slower pace | Faster pace<br>Travel the length of pool |
| 3 minutes | Repeat | | |
| 1 minute | Twist and Jump | Leave out Jump | Mermaids or higher jump |
| 1 minute | Pendulum Push | | Mermaids |

| Table 18.3 (c) | Muscular endurance and low intensity cardiovascular workout with water bells |
|---|---|

**Set up:** Jog in circle to water bells, change direction to resist eddy currents. Find space and perform. On completion, Jog in circle to return water bells.

| Music Counts | Exercise | Adaptation | Progression |
|---|---|---|---|
| I minute | Twist and Jump | Leave out Jump | Rebound |
| I minute | Chest Flyes | Half bell out of water | Narrow side of bell at front Stronger push |
| 2 minutes | Repeat | | |
| I minute | Bicep Curls | Alternate arms | Float prone |
| I minute | Tricep Pushdown | One bell | Bells face down for more drag |
| 2 minutes | Repeat | | |
| I minute | Spotty Dog and Alternate Punch Press | | |
| I minute | Abdominal Pull Through | | |
| 2 minutes | Repeat | | |

| Table 18.4 | Post-workout stretch | | |
|---|---|---|---|

**Set up:** Half group at right wall. Half group at left wall.

| Music Counts | Exercise | Adaptation | Progression |
|---|---|---|---|
| 32 | Face wall<br>Kick heels to buttocks<br>Mobilise knees and<br>ROM<br>Front of thigh stretch | Small range of motion<br>Static stretch | Stronger Jog and<br>push water |
| 32 | Static calf stretch | Use partners if pool wall<br>space limited | Foot against wall |
| 16<br>16 | Face on side of pool<br>Jog high knees<br>Static back of thigh<br>stretch<br>One leg | Float leg<br>Hold poolside | Lift leg higher<br>Foot on poolside<br>Lean forwards |
| 16 | Single arm sweeps | Open fingers | Bigger ROM |
| 16 | Side stretch<br>Lean sideways to<br>poolside | | |
| 16 | Static back of upper<br>arm stretch<br>One side | Without movement | With Jog |
| 32 | To face other<br>poolside<br>Kick heels to buttocks | Side Squat to other side<br>of pool for variety | Stronger Jog and push<br>water |
| 32 | Step away from pool<br>Bear Hugs<br>Mobilise shoulders<br>and ROM<br>Chest and middle<br>back stretch | Slower and smaller static<br>stretch | Fuller ROM |

| Table 18.5 | Mind and body relaxation | | |
|---|---|---|---|
| **Music Counts** | **Exercise** | **Adaptation** | **Progression** |
| | Neutral spine | | |
| | Floating arms | Slice | Fingers closed |
| | Spine twists | Slice | Fingers closed |
| | Push water stabilise | Slice | Fingers closed |
| | Jog knees<br>Float relax | Smaller range<br>Use woggle under arms and knees. With or without partner pulll | Larger range |

# REFERENCES AND RECOMMENDED READING

American College of Sports Medicine (2000) 6th Edition. *Guidelines for Exercise Testing and Prescription.* USA. ACSM.

American College of Sports Medicine (2006) 7th Edition. *Guidelines for Exercise Testing and Prescription.* USA. ACSM.

Bassey, E. and Fentam, P (1981). *Exercise. The facts* UK. Oxford University Press.

Bean, A (1996) 2nd ed. *The Complete Guide to Sports Nutrition* UK. A & C Black.

Borg, G.V (1998) Psychophysical Basis of Perceived Exertion. *Medicine and Science in Sports and Exercise.* Journal 14 (5) (pp. 377–381).

Bursztyn, P.(1990) *Physiology for Sports People. A user's guide to the body.* Manchester University Press.

Davis, D, Kimmet,T and Auty. M (1986) Physical Education Theory and Practice. Australia. MacMillan Education Australia PTY Ltd.

Davis, Roscoe, Roscoe, Bull (2005) Physical Education and the Study of Sport (US. Mosby)

Dinan, S. and Mowbray, L (1988). *Central London YMCA Teacher Training Manual for the Teaching of Exercise for the Older Adult.* UK. CYMCA.

Department of Health (2004). *At Least Five a Week. Evidence on the impact of physical activity and its relationship to health.* A report from the Chief Medical Officer. London. Department of Health.

Department of Health (2005). *Choosing Activity: A Physical Activity Action Plan.* London. Department of Health.

Difiore, J (2003) 2nd ed. *The Complete Guide to Ante-/Postnatal Exercise.* UK. A & C Black.

Fleck, S and Kraemer, W (1987) *Designing Resistance Training Programs.* USA. Human Kinetics.

Fox, E (1984) *Sports Physiology* USA. Saunders College Publishing.

Hall, J (1994) *Physiology of Immersion.* Keynote speech. UK. N.O.W.F.I.T. Aqua conference.

Hazeldine, R (1985) *Fitness for Sport.* UK. The Crowood Press.

Huey, L. and Forster, R (1993) *The Complete Waterpower Workout Book.* Random House.

Krasevec, J. and Grimes, D (1995) *HydroRobics.* Leisure Press.

Lawrence, D (2005) *The Complete Guide to Exercising Away Stress.* UK. A&C Black.

Lawrence, D and Hope, B (2007) 2nd Edition. *Circuit Training: a complete guide to planning and instruction* London. A & C Black.

Lawrence, D and Barnett, L (2006). *GP Referral Schemes.* London. A&C Black.

McArdle, W, Katch, F & Katch, V (1991) *Exercise Physiology. Energy, Nutrition and Human Performance.* USA. Lea and Febiger.

McNeill Alexander, R (1992) *The Human Machine.* UK. Natural History Museum Publications.

Midtlying, J (1988) *National Survey of Water Exercise Participants.* USA. University of Muncie, Indianapolis.

Mitchell, L (1987). *Simple Relaxation. The Mitchell Method for Easing Tension.* UK. John Murray.

Norris, C (1997) *Abdominal Training.* UK. A & C Black.

Norris, C (1994) *Flexibility, Principles & Practice.* UK. A & C Black.

Palmer, M (1988) *The Science of Teaching Swimming* UK. Pelham Books.

Reid Campion, M (1990) *Adult Hydrotherapy.* Heinemann Medical Books.

Smith, H. ed (1968) *Introduction to Human Movement.* USA. Addison-Wesley.

Sova, R (1990) *Aquatics.* USA. Jones and Bartlett Publishing.

Stone, R and Stone, J (1990) *Atlas of the Skeletal Muscles.* USA. Wm Brown Publishers.

Thompson, C (1985) *Manual of Structured Kinesiology.* USA. Times Mirror/Mosby.

Tyldesley, B & Grieve, J (1989) *Muscles, Nerves and Movement.* UK. Blackwell Science Publications

Woodham, A.(1995) *Beating Stress* at Work. UK. Health Education Authority

# USEFUL ADDRESSES

## Training organisations

### Advance Resources and Training Limited
DebbieLLawrence@aol.com

### ASA (Amateur Swimming Association)
Education Department
18 Derby Square
Loughborough LE11 5AL
01509 618722

### YMCA Fitness Industry Training
111 Great Russell Street
London WC1B 3BR
020 7343 1850

## Awarding bodies

### Central YMCA Qualifications
112 Great Russell Street
London WC1B 3NQ
020 7343 1800

## Insurance

### Fitness Professionals
107–113 London Road,
London E13 0DA
0990 133 434
Education@Fitpro.com

## Music

### Solid Sound UK Ltd
PO Box 5978
Laindon, Basildon
Essex SS14 0WD
01268 5488899
info@solidsounduk.com

### Pure Energy Ltd
Hawthorne House
Fitzwilliam Street
Parkgate, Rotherham
South Yorkshire S62 6EP
01709 710022
information@pureenergy.co.uk

### The PRS Foundation
29–33 Berner Street, London W1T 3AB
020 7580 5544

### Phonographic Performance Ltd. (PPL)
1 Upper James Street, London W1R 3HG
020 7534 1000

## Equipment

**The Physical Company Ltd** (supplier of aquatic equipment and workout clothing)
2a Desborough Industrial Park
Desborough Park Road
High Wycombe HP12 3BG
01494 769222
sales@physicalcompany.co.uk

# INDEX